REFERRING THE PSYCHIATRIC PATIENT

Publication Number 878

AMERICAN LECTURE SERIES®

A Monograph in

The BANNERSTONE DIVISION *of*
AMERICAN LECTURES IN CLINICAL
PSYCHIATRY

Edited by

GORDON L. MOORE, M.D.
Department of Psychiatry and Clinical Psychology
Mayo Clinic
Rochester, Minnesota

REFERRING THE PSYCHIATRIC PATIENT

A GUIDE FOR THE PHYSICIAN

By

LARRY R. KIMSEY, M.D.

Clinical Assistant Professor of Psychiatry
The University of Texas
Southwestern
Medical School at Dallas

and

JEAN L. ROBERTS, M.D.

Clinical Instructor of Psychiatry
The University of Texas
Southwestern
Medical School at Dallas

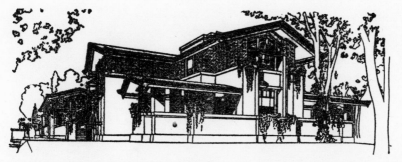

CHARLES C THOMAS • PUBLISHER
Springfield • Illinois • U.S.A.

Published and Distributed Throughout the World by
CHARLES C THOMAS • PUBLISHER
BANNERSTONE HOUSE
301-327 East Lawrence Avenue, Springfield, Illinois, U.S.A.

© *1973*, by CHARLES C THOMAS • PUBLISHER
ISBN 0-398-02725-0
Library of Congress Catalog Card Number: 72-92171

Printed in the United States of America
A-2

FOREWORD

Gordon L. Moore

Doctors Kimsey and Roberts have produced a monograph of significant practical value. With refreshing candor they have dealt with the interprofessional conflict that psychiatry seems to engender. Unfortunately the referral of the psychiatric patient becomes the focal point of physician-psychiatrist controversy. Hence, the person who should be the recipient of the most concern by the professionals involved often is the one who ultimately loses the most because the professionals who are trying to help him cannot seem to understand each other. The authors wisely note that there are several contributions to this difficulty. They provide practical and concrete information about psychiatry and the mechanics of referral. However, they also delve into the prejudices and resistances of all who are involved in this drama—the psychiatrist, the referring physician and the patient. I think all physicians in clinical medicine (including psychiatrists) who find the referral of the psychiatric patient less than a satisfactory experience, would profit from reading this clear, direct and honest book.

PREFACE

W HAT IS THERE ABOUT psychiatry that makes a monograph like this necessary? Is it a field of medicine so different from all the others that special guidelines are needed? Is it so different that physicians and psychiatrists need to be told how to talk with one another? We know of no book entitled *Referring the Thoracic Surgery Patient* or *Referring the Dermatological Patient*. We hear few complaints from doctors concerning their dealings with their nonpsychiatric colleagues. However, we hear many complaints regarding their often frustrating efforts to get psychiatric help for their patients.

We propose that psychiatry is, in a number of significant ways, different from other medical specialties. It is precisely these differences that make it valuable to its patients, but at the same time present a potential for interprofessional friction. What these differences are and how they can be successfully dealt with constitute the subject matter of this monograph.

Mysticism and magical thinking surround the practice of psychiatry—partly due to misconceptions of the public and the nonpsychiatric physician and partly furthered by an "apartheid" on the part of the psychiatrist. What is the reasonableness of being set apart from one's fellow practitioner? It is easy to remember one's residency where calls are received from residents of the other specialties to "get rid of" problem patients occupying bed-space on the medical or surgical wards of the hospital by commitment to a psychiatric institution or certifying the patient will not attempt suicide so that "sick" people may be admitted. Remembrances of being castigated as "non-scientific" return along with the guilt of not being able to pinpoint microscopically a patient's intrapsychic "hang-ups" according to the medical model. Suggesting that mental illness does not obey Koch's postulates usually does not alleviate the psychiatrist's guilt nor inspire understanding and trust on the part of the nonpsychiatric physician.

In fairness, one also remembers wearing a coat and tie and having clean hands and a reasonably well-ordered life while watching the surgical resident in a dirty, bloody scrub suit labor according to the same medical model in an effort to save a patient's life.

There is a growing body of evidence in the psychiatric literature pertaining to the identity crisis of the first-year psychiatric resident.[13,15] This literature describes vividly how the resident, who has spent several years in medical school developing his professional identity, is cast into a strange role of trying to be a physician in an area where paraprofessional people know more about the treatment of the patient than he. How he reacts to the confusion of his new role and the frequent lack of understanding of his nonpsychiatric colleagues has been extensively reported, and the tendency for the psychiatrist to withdraw into his own professional shell is understandable even if not desirable. Appellations of scorn and disdain from his colleagues of other specialties are sometimes defended against by the psychiatrist assuming a quasi-intellectual and philosophical stance to protect his own ego against the strangeness and unfamiliarity of the psychiatrist's medical role.

There is no question that the psychiatrist is a constant reminder to the public and the nonpsychiatric physician of the fact that all of us have emotional "hang-ups." The patient often seems less anxious at confronting the cancer surgeon than the psychiatrist. Impending referral to a psychiatrist frequently has societal overtones of lack of moral fiber, deficiency of willpower, or weakness in one's personality. Fear of psychosis and strangeness keep many patients from the specialized care they need.

That there is a need for psychiatric and nonpsychiatric physicians to work more closely is evidenced by a relatively large amount of literature concerning psychiatric consultation, both for psychiatrists and nonpsychiatrists. Consultation to the other specialties is a part of many psychiatric residency training programs. Adding to the confusion for the nonpsychiatrist are the paramedical professionals associated with most psychiatric programs: social workers, sociologists, the various categories of psychologists, and psychiatric nurses. Additionally, psychiatry has, of necessity, involved itself with economics, political science, anthropology, and archeology in order to understand societies, past and present, as well as our changing social structure as related to mental illness. To be sure, psychiatry is in some ways more closely aligned to the social sciences than to medicine.

Recent advances in psychiatric medicine of a more "scientific" nature should help reassure medicine in general of psychiatry's roots in science and its heritage in physiology and anatomy. The current interest in the limbic system and neuroanatomy and neurophysiology in general, Axelrod's Nobel prize-winning work in neuro-hormonal mechanisms, various animal studies related to aggression, the physiology of mothering, and interest in the physiological and anatomical concomitants of the affects are further proof of psychiatry's concerns with the total personality—uniting *psyche* and *soma* once again as a binary concept for research, teaching, and treatment.

In this monograph, we have tried to resist the "cook-book" approach to the problem, relying instead on many years' experience in general practice, internal medicine, military medicine, teaching medical students and psychiatry residents, and treating a good many patients which involved intimate contact with referring physicians. Thus, we have been on all sides of the psychiatric referral problem and hope to impart some of our perceptions regarding its vicissitudes to both the nonpsychiatric physician as well as to medical students and psychiatric residents in general. If it can serve, in even a small measure, to bridge the gap between the nonpsychiatric physician and the psychiatric specialist, who both strive to bring about better patient care and alleviate hurt and suffering, then our efforts have been well worthwhile.

ACKNOWLEDGMENTS

T HE AUTHORS WISH to express their appreciation to their spouses for their encouragement and support in the writing of this monograph and the authors' previous joint research in geropsychiatry. They also are appreciative of the advice and help from their colleagues at Timberlawn in the formative work on this monograph. Lastly, but of major importance, the authors are grateful to Mrs. Linda Ammons who typed the manuscript, and to Dr. Gordon L. Moore, their editor, whose advice, counsel, and support was a significant factor in the monograph becoming a finished product.

INTRODUCTION

Reports that the generalist and the internist see the vast majority of patients with emotional problems are legion. That these patients make up a large percentage of the practitioner's workload seems indisputable.[12] It also seems appropriate and proper that the general physician, internist, pediatrician, and obstetrician should render the majority of such care inasmuch as they know and are known by the patient, have the patient's trust and confidence, are frequently familiar with the patient's family, work, and life situations, and are by training adept at dealing with most of the emotional and psychological problems that arise from time to time in the lives of their patients. Also, more sophisticated drugs, such as antipsychotic, antidepressant, and antianxiety preparations are readily at their disposal. Medical schools are beginning to increase the proficiency of physicians at understanding psychodynamic constellations in their patients, and thus physicians are more aware of the social-psychological factors involved in the vicissitudes of everyday life.

That the nonpsychiatric physician can and should counsel, advise, prescribe, and treat his patients' psychological maladaptations is not at issue. Indeed, one of the psychiatrist's roles is furthering the psychological skills of his nonpsychiatric colleagues through the process of continuing education in this specialized field.

There are, however, some patients whom the nonpsychiatric physician will, for one reason or other, desire to refer for more specialized psychiatric consultation. We have, therefore, for consideration of the scope of this monograph, chosen to refer to these patients as "psychiatric patients," excluding patients with emotional problems who are treated by their nonpsychiatric physicians. This arbitrary division is more real than apparent and has deep psychological implications for the referral process. Labelling is, unfortunately, a propensity of the patient as well as the physician. The pregnant woman does not object to being her general practitioner's "OB patient." Neither does the patient with a myocardial infarction feel opprobrium in being his internist's "heart patient." We know of no instance where a patient has referred to himself as his GP's "psychiatric patient." The other labels do not cause concern and consternation on the part of either referrent or patient, but the label "psychiatric patient" is frequently a source of discomfort if not outright displeasure. The actual referral is often avoided by avoiding the labeling. Perhaps a good many more years of experience and sophistication will be necessary before this discomfort will not need to be dealt with. In any event, this is one of the unpleasant facts of professional medical life, and it is of the utmost importance in the referral process. How the physician deals with this delicate issue is likely to be of paramount importance in seeing that his patient receives appropriate and skilled care, and it will be dealt with in greater detail in a subsequent chapter.

The physician is frequently troubled and confused in selecting his patients for psychiatric referral. As we have seen, he is eminently capable of managing the majority of his patients with emotional problems. Another reality is the fact that there are only some 18,225 psychiatrists who are members of the American Psychiatric Association, not nearly enough to evaluate all the patients with emotional problems, much less treat them. To compound the problem further, many of these psychiatrists are on medical school faculties, in the armed forces, or assigned to the Veterans' Administration Hospitals and thus, are generally unavailable to the general physician. We shall try to present a schema for determining which patients the physician will need and want to refer to the psychiatrist and how he may best go about the referral process.

Since World War I, a plethora of psychiatric techniques, theories, schools of thought, and facilities have appeared to further confuse the issue. The inception of the National Institute of Mental Health, the Community Mental Health Centers Act, the National Association for Mental Health, the President's Commission on the Mental Health of Children, and others have served to focus public attention on psychiatry and the behavioral sciences. Perhaps psychiatry has promised too much, or the public expects miracles. In any event, a revolution has occurred in America's mental health programs and the resultant confusion has served to muddle, in the minds of many, what may be expected from mental health care resources. In Chapter III, we will attempt a cursory outline of the types of facilities available to the physician and his patients, and in Chapter II, what treatment procedures are generally utilized.

The nonpsychiatric physician, then, faces a dilemma in regards to the psychiatric referral which might appropriately be posed through a series of questions by a hypothetical physician:

"Granted, I know I offer psychological care for most of my patients, and I am aware that most of my patients have psychological disorders, either resulting in symptoms or resulting from the anxiety associated with physical illness. How, then, do I determine from my own practice which patient I refer for psychiatric consultation and how do I devise a reasonable system for considering the various psychiatric disorders?"

"There are so many psychiatric disorders that the American Psychiatric Association has its own diagnostic manual (DSM-II). Is there any way I can systemetize my thinking in this complex area so that I may make a knowledgeable referral?"

"Due to confusion in psychiatric treatment modalities, both somatic and non-somatic, what are some of the things I may expect in the way of treatment for the patients I refer?"

"In addition to there being many treatment modalities, there have been instituted many different sources of psychiatric consultation and treatment. Is there a way that I may understand what each of these facilities offers so that I may best help my patient by making a professionally competent referral?"

"When I have determined which patient needs psychiatric referral and have decided which facility seems appropriate for the patient, what does the psychiatrist or the psychiatric facility require of me in the referral process?"

"Inasmuch as I have a continuing interest in the patient before, during, and after the referral, it is professionally necessary for me to remain informed about the patient. What do I have a right to require and expect from the psychiatrist or psychiatric facility to which I have referred my patient?"

This monograph, then, while not proclaiming itself to be a textbook of psychiatry nor attempting to consider in depth psychodynamics, diagnosis, or psychiatric treatment, will attempt to delineate that very necessary but emotion-charged relationship of physician to physician as evinced through the referral process. This relationship is not peculiar to the psychiatric referral, but because of the very nature of its psychological import, it is frequently subject to misunderstanding, misrepresentation, and misconception. It is dedicated to the mutual respect, understanding, and clear professional communication that is necessary to the physician to physician relationship, and it is predicated on the assumption that both are basically governed by a deep concern for the welfare and well-being of their mutual patient.

CONTENTS

REFERRING THE PSYCHIATRIC PATIENT

---Chapter I---

SELECTING THE
PATIENT FOR REFERRAL

IN THE INTRODUCTION, we noted that, quite appropriately, the nonpsychiatric physician treats most of the patients who present him with psychological complaints. We arbitrarily separated these patients from "the psychiatric patient," the patient who is ultimately referred for more specialized psychiatric evaulation and/or treatment. This was not done to denigrate the psychiatric patient or his physician, but merely to demarcate clearly the treatment situation and take cognizance of the rather specialized techniques necessary for making the referral and the fact that it should be clearly understood by the nonpsychiatric physician that society often looks opprobriously upon psychiatric treatments.

Rather than entering upon a list of psychiatric diagnostic entities and their individual treatment problems, which is beyond the scope of this monograph, we are attempting to separate the classifications of psychiatric syndromes into a more utilitarian concept that might lend itself to a more functional approach for the referring physician. We have chosen to look at the psychiatric referral from the standpoint of a heirarchy of personality disintegration factors, realizing such a continuum exists from necessity among many individual psychiatric diagnostic entities, and that many shades and gradations will readily be apparent to the physician. We have, thus, looked upon the crucial referral point as one of urgency versus elective intervention.

1

Let it be said from the outset that we believe the proper referral consists of any patient with whom the referring physician feels he needs professional help, regardless of the reason for that need. The referring physician is in the front line of defense against physical and mental illness, and it ill-behooves the psychiatric consultant to view or react judgmentally toward the referring physician or his patient. Both referring physician and consultant have obligations to themselves, each other, and the patient; these obligations will be discussed in detail in Chapters IV and V.

The Urgent Referral

The urgency of the referral is almost always predicated upon the assumption that there is some threat to human life, either by possible suicide or homicide. A member of our staff recently remarked that it seemed all referrals were emergencies, meaning that the patient, the patient's family, or his referring physician wanted the patient seen immediately. While prompt attention is often desirable, it is frequently more of a fantasy than an attainable goal due to long waiting periods in many clinics and the general shortage of psychiatrists.

The physician should familiarize himself in advance with the laws of his particular state and the emergency help available to him, for when the emergency arises there is seldom time for such research. It is a fact of medical life that most emergencies arise at inconvenient and inopportune times—particularly nights and weekends. Murders and suicides frequently occur on Saturday and Sunday nights following family arguments and consumption of alcohol. Freud's remark that weekends were the sexualized days of the week could, perhaps, be amended to read "sexualized and aggressivized."

Under such circumstances it is often difficult, if not impossible, to locate an individual psychiatrist, even in this day of answering services and emergency communication systems. In any event, what is needed is not necessarily an individual psychiatrist, but "Help," and help in terms of the institutionalized community services at the physician's disposal. If violence, either homicidal or suicidal, has actually been attempted, what is needed is not psychiatric consultation but definitive medical or surgical care to remove as quickly and effectively as possible the threat to the patient's life. Thus, the general hospital properly receives the bulk of such emergency referrals. A lacerated wrist, a self-inflicted gunshot wound, an overdose of barbiturates are not psychiatric emergencies, but are medical and surgical emergencies, and they must be dealt with before considering definitive psychiatric consultation. Some hospitals make it their practice to admit all suicide attempts and gestures to the psychiatric service. This is of questionable value because psychiatric residents in general are not so adept at suturing wounds, maintaining electrolyte balance, and observing the glomerular filtration rate as are other physicians.

By the same token, other hospitals require that all such patients be seen by the psychiatrist prior to discharge. This is equally as bad as putting all such patients on the psychiatric service initially, because the consultant becomes merely one who certifies that the patient is or is not likely to repeat that act and has little to do with long-term medical management decisions.

Somewhere in between these two extremes lies an area where the psychiatric consultant can function as a member of the health care delivery team and assist other members of the team in devising sound physiological and psychological judgments designed to treat the patient as a total person.

Contemplated homicide or suicide, then, become *bona fide* psychiatric emergencies. Again, while the physician is interested in psychiatric consultation, he is more desirous of getting his patient to a place of safety. He must do this by whatever legal means are at his disposal. If possible, interested family members or friends should be enlisted to share the responsibility with the physician. The police, fire, or sheriff's departments must be notified when the physician is unable to persuade the patient to undertake voluntarily the responsibility of presenting himself for medical care.

In our experience, the vast majority of patients, no matter how emotionally disturbed or agitated, will submit to hospital care if the family and physician courteously but firmly insist on the seriousness of the situation and evidence their determination to procure all legal help possible for the patient. By this, we do not recommend that the physician engage in restraining actions or other overt physical remonstrances with the patient, as the physician is generally not suited by training for physical combat, except to protect himself, which is seldom necessary. If he does engage combatively with the patient, he is likely to be hurt, which is not helpful to himself and is certain to be the subject of much guilt for the patient after he recovers his composure. In any event, those trained for such physical procedures are the police and fire departments. We do not, by the same token, recommend heroics to any physician, as physicians do get killed. Physicians are not paid to take lethal chances, but rather to stay alive and render professional assistance to their patients according to their individual training.

The physician should not be fearful of ascertaining directly from the patient his feelings about violence and his perceptions of how well he is in control of his impulses. Such questioning likely will not cause impulsive behavior on the part of the patient, if properly put, but usually will serve to inform the patient that his physician is aware of the terrible feelings and impulses with which he is contending. Such information and empathy from the physician may serve to quiet the patient and make him more amenable to medical help.

As is not surprising from the foregoing discussion, no mention has been made of diagnostic entities, as they are of little importance initially in the urgent referral situation. The student of such behavior, however, will be interested to know that included on a list of diagnoses which possibly will result in such destructive behavior are agitated depression (neurotic, psychotic, manic-depressive, or schizo-affective), schizophrenia (particularly the paranoid type), alcoholic states, delirium, certain sociopathic states, or the drug-induced psychoses.

To summarize, in the instance of the urgent psychiatric referral, the physician should seek the quickest way possible so as not to endanger his patient or himself. The quickest way will usually not involve the psychiatric consultant but will often necessitate the help of the patient's family or friends, the use of the available municipal resources and the nearest general hospital emergency service. Only later, but hopefully not too much later, will he desire to involve the psychiatric consultant in total planning for the patient's well-being. The saving of human life where possible is the physician's primary responsibility and long-range medical planning his secondary goal.

The Elective Referral

The urgent psychiatric referral requires of the physician promptness, speed, decisive implementation of the "automatic" skills that he has developed through years of practice and experience, and the unhesitant use of emergency community resources. On the other hand, the elective referral requires an entirely different set of abilities—thoughtful contemplation, diagnostic skill, a sure use of the "art of medicine," and a knowledge of the available psychiatric facilities and techniques.

An incomplete list of psychiatric disorders is offered as generally appropriate for referral on an elective basis. Referral facilities are discussed in Chapter III. The physician may desire to add to or delete these psychiatric entities from his own list, depending on his inclination and training. He is referred to any modern textbook of psychiatry for descriptions of the various syndromes.

The Psychoneuroses: The psychoneuroses were, fortunately, the original area of work by Freud, inasmuch as they proved frequently amenable to his psychoanalytic techniques. In a day of societally-sanctioned impulsiveness, the "pure" neuroses as described by Freud are seen with less and less frequency. Nevertheless, they are often debilitating to the patient and can, with some frequency, be successfully treated by the psychoanalyst and psychoanalytically-oriented psychotherapist. Conversion hysteria is almost certainly an overriding indication for psychiatric referral. The phobic may benefit from psychotherapy or the newer behavioral conditioning techniques. The full-blown obsessive-compulsive neurosis is difficult, at best, to treat and often requires years of psychoanalytic treatment with, perhaps, minimal results.

Psychosomatic Disorders: Following the first flush of enthusiasm in the '40's and '50's for the psychiatric treatment of the various pyschosomatic disorders, psychiatrists in general have, in most instances, recognized that such conditions require time-consuming, expensive, and by no means always successful treatment. Also, such disorders often have life-threatening complications which may be exacerbated by the very therapy designed to help them. Therefore, management of these disorders is usually left to the surgeon, internist, and dermatologist. If the psychiatrist decides to attempt treatment of a psychosomatic disorder, he will usually require one of the aforementioned specialists to be available to deal medically or surgically with the complications. On the other hand, a psychiatrist may be useful in consultation to the medical or surgical specialist when considering the overall treatment program. Needless to say, the vegetative expression of psychological conflicts is of much interest to the psychiatrist, and considerable research is continuing; however, it is fair to say that our psychodynamic understanding to date has not led to any treatment breakthrough which would be beneficial to the patient.

The Psychoses: For several centuries, the treatment of the various psychoses has been the *sine qua non* of the psychiatrist. Perhaps psychiatry has made its greatest advances in this area. With the advent of Delay and Deniker's report on the treatment of schizophrenia with the phenothiazines, mental hospital statistics indicate a decline in total hospitalized patients. Indeed, many patients now live in society who would have formerly been condemned to a life of institutionalization. To date, however, no drug has "cured" a patient of schizophrenia, only controlled his symptoms and thus helped him to function in society.

There is no satisfactory treatment for simple schizophrenia, only institutionalization and slow progressive deterioration. The prognosis of paranoid schizophrenia is poor at best with each succeeding episode responding less completely to the chosen treatment program. The manic phase of manic-depressive psychosis is amenable to control by lithium compounds, but the etiology remains in doubt.

The physician will usually desire to refer the psychotic patient for psychiatric evaluation and treatment. The depressive psychosis and the involutional psychotic reaction can be definitively helped. The schizophrenic can often be controlled in his disease process. However, after the initial diagnosis and management procedures are instituted, it often is necessary for the primary physician to maintain the patient's treatment program for a prolonged period of time. He may prefer to do so with psychiatric consultation, but nevertheless it will usually fall his lot to see the patient through his illness for a very long time.

Behavior Disorders: As society has encouraged and sanctioned the expressions of impulses by its members, psychiatrists have seen a turning from the psychoneurosis to the "impulse character," implying a change from problems of conscious affective discomfort to aberrant impulse discharge in the form of delinquency, criminality, sexual promiscuity, and drug and alcohol addiction. Sociopathic and impulsive behavior are, thus, on the increase, and few effective psychiatric techniques have been devised to cope with these disorders. What techniques have been utilized are usually in conjunction with hospitals and law-enforcement agencies. Although society is currently paying the price for these disorders, treatment is most unsure. The physician will often desire advice from his psychiatric consultant relative to the placement of these unfortunate people.

Counseling Problems: Frequently, the physician desires psychiatric consultation relative to certain specific interpersonal disharmonies which are brought to his office. These include marital counseling, job counseling, childrearing problems, and others. Some psychiatrists are adept at counseling techniques, while others will refer the patients to more specially trained psychologists and social workers for such professional help. Certainly, the psychiatrist may be useful in evaluating and helping with the further referral of these patients for more definitive help.

Psychiatric Nomenclature

Perhaps a further word about psychiatric diagnosis is in order. The American Psychiatric Association through the years has expended considerable effort in trying to make nosological sense out of psychiatric nomenclature. Adolf Meyer, a contemporary of Freud, was the most eminent American psychiatrist of the early twentieth century. He devised a system which he called *Psychobiology*. He theorized that the human should be viewed as a unit consisting of both psychological and biological properties which, together and in reaction to environmental stresses and vicissitudes, produced characteristic responses in the organism which he then classified according to these responses or reactions. He felt that mental illness and character formation were the sum total of these reactions which, taken together, succeeded in molding the person's habitual reaction-response. Meyer's great contribution consisted of emphasizing the total psychobiological unit, the unitarian concept of the *psyche* and the *soma* being inseparable and mutually influential. This thinking permeated American psychiatry and resulted in the publication by the American Psychiatric Association in 1952 of the *Diagnostic and Statistical Manual* which was a descriptive compendium of psychiatric diagnostic nomenclature. These diagnoses were heavily weighted in favor of the theory of psychobiological reaction and resulted in such diagnoses as neurotic depressive reaction, schizophrenic reaction, hysterical conversion reaction, and so on. This theory, then, was predicated on the assumption that the human, a psychobiological unit, reacted to environmental stress and produced certain emotional states. While it avoided a consideration of the instinctual theory, it did have much influence on psychiatry rejoining the mainstream of medicine. Unfortunately, as is so common in psychiatry, Meyer felt the need to devise a new terminology to describe these reactions. Such terms as *Ergasia* and *Para-ergasia* temporarily found their way into psychiatric usage, but rather quickly were discarded.

Most of psychiatric diagnosis is difficult to define because these so-called disease states defy examination by the usual scientific criteria, and thus are objectively determined by what appears to most as nonscientific methods. In order to clarify further our qualification of these diagnoses, the American Psychiatric Association appointed a task force to study systematically these diagnoses in an attempt to bring them more closely into approximation with modern psychiatric thinking about the neuroses and psychoses and, at the same time, attempt some correlation between American and (in essence) European psychiatric terminology. The result of the long labor of this task force was the *Diagnostic and Statistical Manual,* 2nd Edition, of 1968 (DSM-II). DSM-II effectively did away with *Reactions* except in the instance of psychotic depressive reaction. The Freudian theory of psychoneurosis was emphasized, bringing a consideration of instinct theory into a perspective consistent with current psychiatric and psychoanalytic thinking and teaching. Thus, we have diagnoses of phobic neurosis, depressive neurosis, anxiety neurosis. Further revision in personality diagnoses also complicated the picture. These changes have met with mixed reactions on the part of the psychiatric community, and it is likely that continued revision will occur, perhaps resulting in DSM-III, IV, V and so forth. Further refinement and revision are of interest to psychiatrists, but they are perplexing and confusing to psychiatrists and nonpsychiatrists alike.

─────Chapter II─────

A SUMMARY OF MODERN PSYCHIATRIC THERAPIES

T HE PHYSICIAN WHO REFERS A PATIENT for psychiatric evaluation and/or treatment, does so partly because he, like all other doctors, is knowledgeable in some areas of medicine and unfamiliar in others. The purpose of this monograph is to facilitate the psychiatric referral process, not to make psychiatrists out of nonpsychiatrists. Therefore, this chapter's discussion of psychiatric therapies is intended only to provide the kind of information that might make the referring doctor more comfortable in talking with his patient about a proposed referral and also make him better able to utilize his consultant's services by making himself more fully aware of the potentials and limitations of psychiatry.

The various psychiatric therapies available can be divided into somatic and nonsomatic modes of treatment. We shall discuss the somatic treatments first.

Somatic Treatments

Psychotropic Drugs: The past two decades have seen a veritable revolution in the medical management of emotional disorders. Prior to the 1950's, psychiatry's pharmaceutical resources were few, limited largely to the sedatives. Now, the number of psychochemotherapy agents available is enormous; it is even possible there may be too many.

9

Three distinct, totally new categories of medication have been developed—the antipsychotics, the antidepressants, and the anti-anxiety agents. Within each category, new products are being developed and manufactured at a rate so fast that no practitioner, psychiatrist included, can have adequate experience with more than a very small percentage of them.

Antipsychotic Agents: It was in the early 1950's that a group of French scientists offered the world chlorpromazine, the first phenothiazine, a drug which in the succeeding years has certainly justified the enthusiasm it originally evoked. Investigated first as an anesthesia-facilitating agent, its tranquilizing effects were duly noted and promptly explored. What had impressed the Frenchmen was chlorpromazine's capacity to calm without sedating or confusing. Delay and Deniker's pioneering clinical explorations and reportings marked the beginning of the modern era in the treatment of psychoses.

Of the three major groups of psychotropic drugs, the antipsychotic drugs are probably the least effectively used by non-psychiatrists for the psychoses. Their value and effectiveness are now well beyond question. However, the patients who require them are the one group of psychiatric patients who most consistently get referred to the psychiatrist. Thus, the family physician is least familiar with these drugs: their dosage schedule, side effects, supplementary use of anti-Parkinson drugs, etc. And there is no obligation for him to become particularly expert in this area. The obligation, if you will, is with the psychiatrist to provide, as a consultant, any information that the referring doctor needs.

In our experience, when nonpsychiatrists employ the antipsychotic drugs to treat psychoses, they use smaller doses than will really do the job. What is more, because they see so few psychotic patients, and treat even less, one bad experience with side effects, i.e. oculogyric crisis, precipitous hypotension, can really dampen their enthusiasm for the whole category of phenothiazines. It can make them reluctant to employ them at all except in very small amounts to treat anxious, nonpsychotic patients where the results are generally poor; the patient notices the annoying side effects of dry mouth, stuffy nose, lethargy, etc. and does not experience a real release for his anxiety. Phenothiazines are not antianxiety drugs; they are antipsychotic medicines.

Phenothiazines do not cure psychoses. They control the symptoms of psychoses. And they do this with great effectiveness no matter what the precise cause of the disorder, be it toxic delirium, "senile" psychosis, schizophrenic reaction, etc. When the psychosis abates, the phenothiazine medication may be stopped. For those persons suffering from what, for lack of a better term or explanation, is called chronic schizophrenia, a life-long maintenance on medication will be needed, much as a diabetic continues to require insulin. People do not become addicted or habituated to these drugs, but if their psychosis persists, so will the need for symptomatic control remain.

The phenothiazines appear to be the indisputable leaders in the job of controlling psychotic symptoms. Rauwolfia derivatives have been used for this purpose, but they are seldom used in this country at present. Although effective in controlling excitement and agitation, they have the unfortunate capacity to produce depressions.

One new, highly specific, highly successful nonphenothiazine drug is lithium, offered in the form of lithium salts and used to control the manic phase of manic-depressive psychoses. The administration of lithium is a procedure that is most prudently left to those specialists who not only have the knowledge, but the facilities with which to perform very careful laboratory monitoring of the patient's electrolyte balance. Unfortunately the therapeutic dose of lithium is precariously close to the toxic level.

Antidepressants: The antidepressants were discovered close on the heels of the antipsychotics. First there were the MAO inhibitors with their undeniable effectiveness but also their alarming side effect of fatal bursts of hypertension. Then came the development of the tricyclic drugs, and the medical treatment of depression was almost as radically changed as was the treatment of the psychoses by the phenothiazines. The tricyclics have proved to be very effective and relatively safe to use.

It is very probable that referring doctors have as much or more experience with this group of drugs as do many of the psychiatrists to whom they refer patients. In current American living, even highly transient depressive episodes are often viewed as illnesses worthy of treatment rather than as one's temporary lot in life. So, presumably far more persons are presenting themselves to their family doctors for help with depression. In addition more family doctors are becoming aware of the hidden depressions that lie behind many somatic complaints. With so many effective antidepressant drugs available to them, family doctors are treating large numbers of depressed patients pharmacologically. Those depressed persons who get referred to the psychiatrist are, for the most part, either those who appear suicidally or psychotically depressed, or those who fail to respond to the antidepressant drugs. In the latter category, most of the patients are struggling with reactive depressions, that is to say depressions that occur in response to some interpersonal loss or conflict, in which case far better results will be obtained with psychotherapy than with pills. The target symptoms that seem to prognosticate good results with the antidepressant drugs are the classic symptoms of guilt and diminished self-worth in association with symptoms of vegetative disruption, i.e. early morning insomnia and loss of appetite.

Prior to the introduction of the antidepressants, short-acting stimulants such as the amphetamines and Ritalin® were often prescribed. Their effects are almost immediate, compared with the antidepressants which require 10 to 14 days for symptom diminution. As the term stimulant implies, they produce an actual sense of increased energy as opposed to an absence of depression. It has become apparent in recent years that the amphetamines have far too great a potential for abuse to make them a wise medication choice. Even aside from that, they are not really adequate treatment for depressions, because their action is so short-lived, and depressive episodes of suicidal proportions occur not uncommonly as rebound phenomena. Ritalin, though not so widely abused as the amphetamines, does have a proclivity for dependency that the tricyclic antidepressants do not have. Like the amphetamines, its action is prompt and short-lived. It actually has greater usefulness in combating the drowsiness that is occasionally a problem in phenothiazine therapy than it has in the treatment of depressions.

Antianxiety Agents: NIMH recently published the results of three national surveys which substantiated the commonly held impression that most psychotherapeutic drugs are prescribed by nonpsychiatrists, mainly general practitioners and internists, and that the most frequently prescribed category of drugs is the antianxiety agents.[14]

These medications, along with the phenothiazines and the antidepressants also had their beginnings in the 1950's. Meprobamate was probably the first popular drug in this group. Within the past few years it has fallen into some disfavor because of its propensity to produce dependency in those inclined to self-medication.

In marked contrast to the antipsychotic and antidepressant agents, the antianxiety drugs do not have the same degree of clearly proven effectiveness. Thus, any practitioner who appraises one of his anxious patient's requests for help needs to weigh several factors before deciding in favor of prescribing a "tranquilizer." First, there is the always present problem of drug side effects, so that no medication ought be offered lightly and without really good evidence for its need. Secondly, in prescribing a pill for anxiety, one is suggesting that this is the acceptable way to avoid or relieve the rather minor tensions of ordinary daily living. It is our impression that many patients accept a prescription as a substitute for what they are really wanting—a chance to talk to someone.

Convulsive Therapies: The convulsive therapies are treatment methods with which most referring doctors are not personally familiar. Possibly a physician did not witness any "shock treatments" during his medical school and internship days. If he did, perhaps all that remains to him of the experience is the disquieting recollection of the scene of the convulsion itself, with no firm memory remaining regarding the indications for, mechanisms of, and likely outcome associated with the use of this treatment technique.

Therefore, in the sometimes uncomfortable but frequently inevitable role the family doctor plays as liason man between family and patient during a psychiatric hospitalization (or between patient and psychiatrist prior to patient's first meeting with the recommended psychiatrist or psychiatric facility) it might prove helpful to the nonpsychiatrist for us to present a brief discussion of electroconvulsive therapy, the most commonly employed convulsive method and the one frequently (though mistakenly) labelled "electroshock."

Fits have occurred naturally for as far back as we have any way of knowing about. As a treatment device they have been with us since the 1930's, when von Meduna began producing seizures with camphor and later Metrazol®; Sakel began evoking them with insulin, and Cerletti and Bini began obtaining them with alternating electrical current. At the present time, it is only the last mentioned method that continues to be widely used, along with a more recent (1957) method involving hexafluorodiethyl ether inhalation.

Despite the distaste that laity and physicians (many psychiatrists included) seem to have for "shock treatment," and despite the almost miraculous impact that the psychotropic drugs have had on so many forms of mental illness, ECT remains to this day the treatment of choice in involutional melancholia and in any of the other psychotic depressions which do not respond to drugs. It is also frequently useful in some forms of schizophrenia (i. e. catatonic excitement).

ECT, in addition to being highly effective in treating severe depressions, is also notably safe to use. It has been said that it is actually safer, statistically speaking, than any of the psychotropic drugs. Kalinowsky,[5] who is probably the outstanding authority on convulsive treatments, says there is no absolute contraindication to ECT other than brain tumor (where the sudden increase in intracerebral pressure during the seizure can present a real hazard). According to Kalinowsky, the death rate involved in ECT was around 0.1 percent before the procedure was refined by the administration of anesthesic agents prior to giving the muscle relaxant and applying the current. With the advent of the use of anesthesia has come the inherent hazards, but ECT still remains remarkably safe.

Despite its unchallenged effectiveness and its relative safety, ECT remains a treatment method that is not undertaken lightly. Certainly, the laity and nonpsychiatric physicians view it warily. Even among psychiatrists there is a noticeable ambilvalence about it. In some ways, those psychiatrists who are willing to administer it are looked upon in the same way that we view our nation's spies; people doing a job that is seen as necessary but somehow distasteful.

Partly, among psychiatrists, the discomfort that ECT arouses has to do with our ignorance of how it works. Thus, it comes very close in the minds of many to a sort of witchcraft. There is staunch agreement that ECT has no influence on basic personality, nor does it effect any demonstrable pathological or morphological changes. What it does is alleviate depression, and after as few as four treatments.

In trying to make some sense out of how ECT works, it has been suggested by some that the term "electroshock" may not be a misnomer after all. Though the treatment produces a seizure and not a shock, the procedure, very certainly, is viewed as psychologically "shocking" by most everyone, including those who undergo it. It is, for example, well recognized that during a course of ECT, patients rather consistently develop a sense of dread concerning each succeeding treatment. This sense of dread is traditionally seen as ECT's most troubling side effect. And yet, it is proposed by some that the process of undergoing a dreaded experience is the pivotal part of the treatment. A severely depressed person is in many cases, and consistently so in involutional melancholia, a severely guilt-ridden person, someone whose rigid conscience demands self punishment for imagined transgressions. Thus, the assaultive, frightening aspects of ECT may be viewed as proper punishment by the patient who is relieved of his guilt and no longer needs to feel depressed. Another more recent explanation, in keeping with the cybernetics viewpoint, is that ECT "clears the computer," thus wiping away the depression and letting the patient start anew. It may also alter intersynaptic transmissions of nerve impulses.

In summary, ECT is the most effective treatment available for the relief of involutional melancholia and for all other forms of severe depression which do not respond to the antidepressants or in which either suicidal or agitated elements are so great that medication with its slower and less certain effects is deemed likely to be inadequate. It appears to be generally safe and free of long-term side effects. It is also unpleasant; but this criticism can be made of many medical and all surgical procedures.

Lobotomies: The destruction of part of the cerebral pathways to relieve emotional symptoms is undoubtedly the most controversial psychiatric treatment currently available. Interestingly, it was for the development of this technique that Egas Moniz was awarded one of the only two Nobel prizes ever given to psychiatrists. It was in 1936 that he presented to the scientific world a report of the symptom relief twenty psychotic patients had obtained after undergoing surgical destruction of some of their frontal lobe connections. Thanks to Freeman and Watts' enthusiasm for the procedure here in this country, the 1940's became the decade of the lobotomies. Then, with the availability of the phenothiazines in the early 1950's, lobotomies rapidly receded in popularity.

Now there are indications of a resurgence of interest.[3] Newer technical developments have made possible a much greater degree of precision with regard to what is being destroyed,[4] and the means of destruction have certainly become more varied and more sophisticated than was the case back in the days of so called "ice pick" lobotomies. Furthermore, great strides have been made in our understanding of neurophysiology, and this has been reflected in greatly refined theories as to what portions of the brain ought to be tampered with.

Historically, the emotionally calm chimpanzees which first caught Moniz's attention had been rendered tranquil by an actual frontal lobe extirpation. In humans lobe destruction was not employed; it was fiber tract interruption that was used. These days there are a number of specific sites in the brain that are being precisely ablated, each procedure having its own name to describe the specific site of the lesion, i.e. cingulectomy. None of these procedures is psychiatric treatment; they are all neurosurgical operations. And their greatest supporters are neurosurgeons, not psychiatrists. Currently, a remarkably diverse assortment of disorders is being treated in this manner; there are clinical reports of good results in such varied problems as drug addiction, schizophrenia, and frigidity as well as with the classic symptom indication of "agonizing" anxiety.

Another psychosurgical procedure undergoing investigation is the stimulation of particular areas of the brain via deeply placed electrodes. One application of this that seems to have intriguing possibilities is the combating of intractable pain by electrically evoked sensations of intense pleasure.

It is safe to say, the final verdict is not yet in regarding lobotomies or electrode stimulation. It is possible that continued increase in neurophysiological knowledge will sustain and increase the current revival of interest in psychosurgery. However, at present most psychiatrists remain unenthusiastic and critical of lobotomies in general.

Ervin et al[1] at Harvard have elucidated what they call the dyscontrol syndrome, a disorder in which the person is subject to uncontrollable outbursts of destructive rage. They have treated psychosurgically some of these patients, when this syndrome has been associated with intractable epilepsy. Others of these patients, those who are not epileptic, have benefitted by a more traditional medical approach, involving medications and supportive psychotherapy. The Harvard group looks upon the dyscontrol syndrome as an excellent example of the complex interplay between organic, neurological factors and environmental and psychological factors. This would seem to be the most fruitful framework within which to examine and evaluate the whole field of psychosurgery.

Electrosleep: Very new on the American scene but employed by the Russians for a quarter of a century is the somatic treatment popularly called electrosleep.[9] As with electroshock, the term is something of a misnomer. Sleep may or may not occur during the treatment. What does happen, according to proponents of this procedure, is that a disrupted night sleep pattern is restored to a normal sleep pattern, and this restoration is subsequently accompanied by the diminution or disappearance of a number of other psychological symptoms, i.e. anxiety, headache, etc. Thus, a better term for the procedure is transcerebral electrotherapy.

By means of a machine designed especially for this purpose, the patient, while resting comfortably, receives a very weak electrical current (DC) via electrodes placed over his mastoid bones and over his eyes (or on his forehead directly above his eyes). All that the patient experiences physically is a mild tingling at the electrode site. The current is applied for one-half to one hour per treatment. Ten to fifteen of these treatments given daily on a five-day week basis constitute a typical course of treatment.

Precise indications for electrosleep (TCET) have not yet been established. (It may well be that more general practitioners than psychiatrists are currently using it.) A very wide variety of psychological disorders are reported as benefitting from it, but most of these accounts are hard to evaluate being clinical examples rather than experimental studies. Research is underway at present in a number of medical school settings. Not only do we need to know if TCET has a true effectiveness apart from its nonelectrical aspects; if it does do something to the brain, we would like to know what it does and how it does it. Its proponents point to its record in Russia of clinical safety and effectiveness as being a sound basis for present clinical use in this country.

Nonsomatic Psychiatric Treatments

Individual Psychotherapy: Psychotherapy refers to treatment by psychological methods or interventions. Historically, it goes back to the witchcraft of primitive man (just as psychopharmacology goes back to ancient herbs and roots). But our modern versions of psychotherapy have their origins in Sigmund Freud's psychoanalysis.

It was Freud who discovered that psychiatric symptoms have unconscious meanings to their possessor, that the meanings can be shared and understood by others, and that in the sharing and the understanding the symptoms can be given up.

It was at the turn of this century that Freud first conceptualized this. He was then a young neurologist who found himself frustrated by his patients' frequent failures to respond to the somatic treatments that were standards of Viennese medical practice. A fellow physician had caught his attention with the story of a rather remarkable young woman whose numerous somatic symptoms disappeared when she talked about them with her doctor and in the talking relived, emotionally, the actual situations in which they had first occurred. Freud's genius led him to believe that this was not just a chance happening, but that it could work with other patients, too, and that it was his colleague's willingness to assume the more passive listening role that somehow facilitated the patient's symptom removal. With these hunches, Freud set forth on a totally new type of medical practice. And out of the vast amount of clinical experience that he acquired, he wove a whole new system of human psychology and psychopathology. Psychoanalysis, as a specific treatment method, was recognized by him as having limited clinical applications: hysteria, phobias, and obsessive-compulsive neuroses were seen as its only indications. However, psychoanalysis as a science of human psychology has had far wider application. Its two basic tenets, the concept of an unconscious and the concept of psychic determinism, have had an influence on the western world's understanding of human behavior that cannot be overestimated.

Although classical psychoanalysis is still an excellent treatment method for the psychoneuroses, it is not widely applicable because it functions best with the neuroses; it requires a long period of time with a frequency of 4 to 6 visits per week and it is extremely expensive. Modifications have been attempted for the treatment of children and adolescents, the psychoses, and the character disorders. It is, however, extremely useful as a theoretical framework for understanding and teaching psychodynamics, and it is also a useful research tool. Also, psychoanalytic theory and techniques are useful and applicable in psychotherapy.

Only within the past couple of decades has psychotherapy begun to be something other than totally private. With the introduction of one-way viewing screens and video tapes, and perhaps most significantly with the advent of group therapy, it is now possible for a therapist to show others how he works, what he really does. Out of this has come a growing conviction that all effective therapists, no matter what their theoretical persuasion, be they Freudian, Jungian, Alderian, Sullivanian, Rogerian, existential, transactional, gestalt, or whatever, they are more alike than different regarding the way they work with their patients.

The principal tool of the effective therapist seems to be his capacity for creative listening. By his willingness to hear whatever the patient needs to say he helps the patient acquire not only an understanding of himself but also a sense of value about himself and his very human needs. Probably all persons who have sufficient emotional distress to seek psychotherapy are suffering from serious threats to their self-esteem, and their symptoms can be viewed as desperate means to defend against these threats. So the effective therapist is one who listens with respect.

But he obviously does more than listen. Out of his general knowledge of human psychology and out of his specific knowledge of a given patient, the therapist responds in ways designed to increase the patient's understanding of himself. Some of the responses are formulations that the therapist proposes as interpretations of what the patient does, thinks, or feels. Other responses are not explanations but feedback. By feedback we mean the process of informing the patient of the effect he has upon the therapist (and thus presumably upon other people in his life). The idea that he has influence on others around him often comes as a complete surprise to patients in psychotherapy. Most often these people see themselves as weak underlings being acted upon by a hostile and powerful world. Therefore, this feedback-type response can be a great restorative force. The responses of interpretation and feedback are all aimed at clarifying a patient's behavior to himself and helping him find ways, if he then chooses, to change those parts of his behavior that are causing him emotional pain or suffering.

Group Therapy: The past decade or so has seen such a proliferation of treatment techniques that no person (psychiatrist or nonpsychiatrist) can stay abreast of all of them. One major innovation, already cited though not yet discussed, is group therapy. A nonpsychiatric physician named J. H. Pratt is acknowledged as the first to employ this method in America. At the turn of the century in Boston, Dr. Pratt organized his tubercular patients into groups for purposes of explaining to them their illness and the management of it and hence promoting their adequate participation in a home treatment program. It was the military requirements of World War II that brought the first widespread use of this treatment method into psychiatry. The vast numbers of psychiatric casualties and the shortage of military psychiatrists forced the abandonment of the traditional method of individual psychotherapy. Group therapy in America thus began as a wartime expediency. But it was soon recognized by many psychiatrists as having specific therapeutic values of its own, values that individual psychotherapy did not possess. Today it is a highly respected form of therapy, not a second-rate substitute offered when a patient cannot afford to buy an hour all to himself or when the therapist is so busy that he hasn't enough time to see each of his patients separately.

The advantages and the apparent successes of group therapy have led to an enormous proliferation of kinds of groups available. Three major subgroups seem worth mentioning. There is the homogeneous group experience in which persons with a common problem are brought together for information, guidance, and mutual support; one such group might be one comprised of alcoholics. Here, the emphasis is on the handling of current real life situations. The other two major categories of group therapy divide themselves with regard to how they use the group experience to promote the psychical growth of the group members. One is the analytic approach, which comes at times rather close to being individual therapy done in a group setting; that is, emphasis is placed on psychological material brought to the group by the various members (be it dreams, past history, etc.), and this material is reacted to by the other group members. The other approach is an experiential or existential one. Here the focus is on the immediate interactions of the group members with each other and with the group leader. Members are encouraged to express their spontaneous, here-and-now feelings as these feelings develop in the group rather than to bring in accounts of what they have done elsewhere, be it in their dreams, in their past history, or in their current extragroup activities. As one might assume from reading the foregoing, these two approaches are by no means mutually exclusive, and probably most psychiatrists who do group work tend to employ a combination of both orientations.

There is one other specific form of group therapy that ought be mentioned, not because it is so widely used, but because a number of its techniques have found their way into other kinds of therapy groups. We are speaking here of psychodrama, a highly stylized form of group therapy originated in Europe by Moreno. It involves the actual acting out, in the theatrical sense, of a patient's conflicts and feelings. As already mentioned, in its pure form, it is a highly specialized technique, and those therapists who use it need very specific training.

It may be less obvious and therefore important for us to state that to do any type of group therapy does indeed involve specialized training. A group therapist certainly needs to be well trained in psychodynamics and psychopathology. But in addition he needs knowledge of group dynamics and group process. Perhaps even more than the psychiatrist who does only individual work, the group therapist needs a tolerance for and an appreciation of spontaneity, uncertainty, and mutual openness between himself and his patients.

Typically, a therapy group consists of five to ten patients who meet for one ninety-minute session per week. Most groups have one leader; some have co-leaders. As with all psychotherapy, outcome studies are extremely difficult to design, and thus it has been hard to demonstrate the effectiveness of group therapy (or individual therapy for that matter) by any strict scientific studies. Clinically, however, their value seems well-established.

Not to be confused with therapy groups are the "encounter

groups" and "sensitivity groups" that have mushroomed in recent years. Their entire development has been outside the medical domain, and they have addressed themselves to the nonpatient population of our country, people who feel they want to realize their full emotional potential through experiencing the power of group process. Psychiatrists for the most part take a dim view of these groups and for a number of reasons. The leaders of such groups may or may not be competent, anyone who so desires may call himself a group leader. There is usually no screening of group members with the implication that such groups are good for everyone, when in truth they may be highly destructive, and as a rule there are no back-up or follow-up facilities to take care of those psychiatric casualties that may occur.

Milieu Therapy: Milieu therapy is a hospital or day care center type of treatment. It refers to the recognition and utilization of the curative factors inherent in the social structure of the hospital or the day care center. It acknowledges that, in addition to the psychiatrist and the drugs, ECT, or pyschotherapy he may prescribe and deliver, there are many other therapeutic resources available to the patient. We are speaking, of course, of the ancillary services of such trained professionals as the psychiatric nurse, the occupational therapist, the music therapist, the psychiatric orderly, et al. But we are also speaking of the benefits the patient can derive from interacting with the other patients with whom he lives during his hospitalization. It used to be a sad paradox that people who were having such grave discomfort about their own autonomy as to require psychiatric hospitalization were then treated by means that could only further diminish their sense of self-worth. They were regimented, controlled, and institutionalized. The development of milieu therapy has been an attempt to avoid the iatrogenic problems of institutionalization and to turn the same social system into a growth-promoting opportunity. The underlying philosophy has been a desire to have the patient be an active participant in his own treatment program, to take as much responsibility for himself and his hospitalization as he can at any given time, and to learn within the hospital setting the social skills he will need in order to live effectively outside the hospital. Such things as patient-staff ward meetings are an example of milieu philosophy.

Behavior Therapy: Behavior therapy should be mentioned separately because its theoretical framework sets it apart from the various schools of dynamic psychiatry, i.e. those that see unconscious conflict as the basis for psychiatric symptoms. Behavior therapy takes its origins in learning theory and in a sense echoes Adolf Meyer who saw psychopathology as faulty habit patterns rather than collisions between unconscious wishes and prohibitions.

Behavior therapists do not concern themselves with the underlying meaning that a symptom may have for a patient. They direct their efforts toward abolishing, rather than understanding, a symptom, and actually that is what the patient is most desirous of also.

Four particular forms of behavior therapy are receiving increasing clinical application these days. Both desensitization techniques and reciprocal inhibition techniques are reported as being very effective in treating phobias. Conditioned avoidance techniques, long used in treating alcoholism, now are also being successfully employed in treating homosexuality, fetishism, and exhibitionism. For these sexual problems, electrical shocks are used as the aversive stimulus.

A fourth technique, positive reinforcement, does not seek to eliminate a troublesome symptom but rather to evoke a desired behavior. One of its major applications so far has been to improve the social behavior of chronic, hospitalized patients by rewarding them in some very specific way (i.e. coins or candy) each time they display the particular behavior that the staff is wanting them to acquire.

Summary

This chapter has catalogued and briefly described a great many psychiatric therapies. The purpose has been to give the referring physician an awareness of the vast array of help available to those of his patients who need psychiatric treatment. It is not proposed that the physician become expert in any of these procedures or even that he become skilled in deciding which procedure will be most useful to any given patient. Instead, it is proposed that such deciding and implementing is an integral part of the service his psychiatric colleague can offer.

The past decade or so has seen such a proliferation of treatment techniques that no person (psychiatrist or nonpsychiatrist) can stay abreast of all of them. There is the traditional individual therapy, there is group therapy with one leader and group therapy with co-leaders, there is the treatment of a couple by a single therapist and there is the treatment of a couple by a couple. There is even treatment of an individual by multiple therapists.

But within all these various patient-therapist combinations it seems that the common ingredients are an opportunity for the patient really to talk and share his style of behavior with someone who offers receptive listening without control and who can show the patient, without threatening his self-esteem, how he can change those aspects of his feelings and behavior which cause him pain.

Chapter III

SELECTING THE
PSYCHIATRIC FACILITY

W E MENTIONED EARLIER THAT PSYCHIATRY, its practitioners, its ancillary paraprofessional and nonprofessional workers, its facilities, and its various treatment modalities began proliferating after World War II. Not only is psychiatry now the third largest medical specialty in the United States, being exceeded numerically only by medicine and surgery, but it is probably the most confusing specialty due to the myriad ways it delivers its services. If it requires a psychiatry resident three years to come to a fair understanding of how psychiatry delivers its services, how can one expect the nonpsychiatric physician to experience other than confusion?

Real impetus to psychiatry came from World War II and the military experiences with the emotional problems of the servicemen. Following World War II, many physicians put their interest into specializing in psychiatry. With the increase in psychiatric education came increases in psychiatric research and treatment programs. Because of the relative newness of the specialty, numerous individuals struck out in many divergent directions in search of more information. These divergent approaches further compounded the confusion indigenous to a specialty built on abstract thinking.

President Kennedy's health message to Congress which resulted in the Community Mental Health Centers Act of 1963, gave federal

25

impetus to the development of psychiatry. Suddenly, the nation was swept up in an enthusiasm of concern for the mentally ill. Suddenly medical and psychiatric care became a *right* of the people, not a *privilege*. Programs for the poor and indigent were demanded by the federal government. Medical schools and state and local governments were swept into the melee in a frantic effort to stem the tide of mental illness. Early, and perhaps false hopes of a quick solution to the problem arose from Delay and Deniker's 1955 announcement of the effectiveness of the phenothiazines on schizophrenia. In short order, many mental hospitals were emptied. It seemed that all that was needed for "the final solution of the mental health problem" was to spend more and more money. More money was spent. Further less dramatic advances have been made, and psychiatry has become more complex and confusing. Adding to the picture has been the plight of a nation in turmoil. Psychiatrists have been concerned with student unrest, Women's Lib, Black protest, Viet Nam, legal medicine, and psychotomimetic drugs.

Psychiatric research has gone on in many directions, also. Advances have been made in our understanding of the neurohormonal mechanisms of the transmission of nerve impulses and the relation to depression. The outgrowth of this has been the antidepressant medications. Lithium has been shown to be effective in the manic phase of manic-depressive psychosis.

Social concerns have led to research into population masses and the socioeconomic causes and effects of mental illness. Hollingshead and Redlich in their study of the citizens of New Haven showed the diagnosis of schizophrenia was made more often among the deprived, indigent, and lower socioeconomic patients, while obsessive-compulsive neurosis was diagnosed more often in middle and upper class people. On the other hand, Faris and Dunham in Chicago showed that people with schizophrenia "drifted" into the ghetto, suggesting the ghetto was not a causative factor in the origin of the psychosis. The Midtown Manhattan Study and the Stirling County Study further heightened our interest in the demography of mental illness. We are now trying to understand mental illness from an epidemiological standpoint.

Now why is it necessary to discuss, in a monograph such as this, psychiatry's dilemma? Obviously, it is impossible to go into detail in a few pages. It seems important to outline some of the areas of psychiatrists' interests so that the physician will have a flavor of the excitement and flux in which psychiatry currently finds itself. Also, we feel it important to explore, no matter how cursorily, the numerous psychiatric facilities available to the physician, as the facilities spring from the variables discussed in Chapter II and the introduction to this chapter. The physician has a wide variety of psychiatric facilities at his disposal, and if he is reasonably well-informed about what they have to offer his patient, he can make more logical judgments about securing the needed care. We will attempt, then, to summarize the more important psychiatric facilities that the physician may wish to consider when referring the psychiatric patient.

A word must be said about the geographic location of the referring physician. To some extent, the choice of psychiatric facility will be determined by this. Availability of resources differs, for instance, between the highly populated urban areas and the more sparsely populated rural areas. Now, however, accessibility of psychiatric care is no longer the problem it was several years ago. Although a psychiatric facility may not exist in the community of residence of the referring physician, he should not be far from a community mental health center, a VA hospital, or a state psychiatric hospital.

Non-Private Psychiatric Facilities

The following discussion will attempt to encompass a summary of several publicly funded facilities available to the physician for referral of his patients. While there are many similarities and overlapping functions common to these facilities, they, at the same time, have specific functions as defined by law. We have avoided any consideration of the psychiatric functions of the armed forces.

Veterans Administration Hospitals: In general, any person who has been a member of the armed forces of this country, is entitled to medical care at a V.A. hospital. There are some restrictions related to retirement and type of discharge; however, that is beyond the scope of our presentation.

The V.A. provides several types of programs for its psychiatric patients. There are inpatient, outpatient, emergency, and partial hospitalization services available, depending on the facility. The Veterans Administration maintains an office in most major cities for purposes of disseminating information to inquirers. One should call this office for direction. The veteran entitled to V.A. psychiatric care will not be charged for the care, and the psychiatric disability does not have to be service-connected.

As a part of its overall medical program, the V.A. designates certain facilities for the following psychiatric functions: long-term psychiatric care, acute psychiatric care, and domiciliary care. After referral, the V.A. physicians will determine which approach seems most suitable for the patient. Patients may be committed to V.A. hospitals just as they may be committed to other psychiatric facilities.

Community Mental Health Centers: Since the enactment of the Community Mental Health Centers Act in 1963, many areas which once were devoid of any mental health facilities now have community mental health centers nearby. The object of the Act was to provide all citizens with mental health care without regard to cost. Unfortunately, the more remote centers have had problems in securing trained staff, particularly on the psychiatric level. Because of the emphasis on *mental* health, these centers were not set up in conjunction with other health areas; thus *psyche* was once again artificially separated from *soma*. At any rate, more and more people now at least have access to mental health care whereas before a tremendous void existed in this area.

Each center serves a "catchment area" approved by the appropriate section of the Department of Health, Education, and Welfare. All persons residing within the boundaries of the catchment area, regardless of financial status or income, are entitled to care from the center. Admission procedures may be obtained from the office of the director of any center, but suffice it to say, all persons in the area that request evaluation must be seen.

The Act requires each center, in order to be eligible for federal funding, to provide five basic psychiatric services: inpatient, outpatient, partial hospitalization, emergency services, and consultation. Some of these services may be contracted for with other mental health facilities. For instance, it is not uncommon for several community mental health centers to share a common emergency service. Staffing is often partially provided by part-time personnel, such as psychiatrists in private practice who devote a portion of their time to such work. Direct patient care usually is not in the area of intensive individual psychotherapy, but rather intervention may focus on the family, the social group, or the subcommunity. Group psychotherapy, crisis intervention, counseling techniques, psychopharmacological therapy, and family therapy are often used. The social processes which are thought to bring about the patient's maladaptation to life are dealt with by social workers. Environmental change and social action in the areas of jobs, sanitation, malnutrition, and living conditions are routine procedures. Child-rearing practices are concerns of these centers.

The sheer number of patients seeking help from these centers has made innovation a necessity. The weight of these numbers has made it difficult to assay intelligently the effectiveness of this form of mental health intervention. Whatever the outcome, the community mental health centers movement represents the first time in this country that the federal government and a large segment of the population saw the need to act in the area of mental health, and made a significant assault on the problem through a massive health care delivery system approach.

University and Charity Hospitals: Most university teaching hospitals have had psychiatric services for some time. These have often been staffed by full-time teachers who utilize the patient population for purposes of educating medical students and psychiatric residents. Psychiatry wards, inpatient consultation, emergency consultation, and outpatient services have become standard features of such hospitals. While in some instances paralleling the work of the community mental health center program, these university hospitals have, in other instances, because of their emphasis on training and research, been able to give the individual patient more of an in-depth treatment approach. Intensive, individual psychotherapy, longer-term hospitalization, intensive group and family psychotherapy are much more common than in the community mental health center. Staffing problems are often not so acute inasmuch as the medical school may be able to attract competent people because of intellectual interests and the opportunity of research. University psychiatric services have increased their staffs as the medical schools have become more aware of the need to teach medical students psychological principles and terminology as well as treatment procedures.

Although psychiatric services have not been strangers to university hospitals, it is a fairly recent development that charity hospitals, and by this we mean county and city hospitals unassociated with medical schools, have undergone significant changes in their approach to the mental patient. While many still function in the psychiatric areas as holding and/or evaluation centers for psychiatric patients, or as emergency centers for dealing with severe emotional upheavals, many of these hospitals are more recently developing full-fledged psychiatric services offering both inpatient and outpatient services. They are discovering the value of rotating house staff through the psychiatric service as a means of broadening the intellectual and affective scope of the young intern or resident. Here again, we find psychiatry too long separated and segregated from its sister specialties. The large, reasonably well-staffed charity hospital is often eminently capable of offering a well-rounded psychiatric service to its patients.

State Psychiatric Hospitals and Clinics: The seeds of psychological medicine in this country grew from the efforts of the various state psychiatric institutions. The American Psychiatric Association had its antecedents in the Association of Medical Superintendents of American Institutions for the Insane, organized in 1844, and antedating the American Medical Association by a good many years. This association was instrumental in helping the early psychiatrists form and maintain their identities as medical pyschologists in an alien environment.

The state hospitals account for a large proportion of total hospitalized psychiatric patients in this country. They generally serve a specified area of their state, and they receive many patients through legal commitment. Commitment proceedings vary somewhat from state to state, but generally a patient is committed, when he refuses voluntary admission after he is adjudged by the court as being a danger to himself or others.[6]

Because of the large numbers of patients admitted to these state hospitals and the frequent disparity in staff-patient ratio, intensive individual psychotherapy is infrequently utilized because of problems of time. The somatic therapies and psychopharmacology are heavily relied upon. Also, reliance on milieu therapy, ward management procedures, patient government, token economies, conditioning techniques, and various forms of therapeutic pressure through peer group interactions are utilized. Less completely trained personnel such as psychiatric aides, volunteers, and BA-degree psychologists are often used to help fill the gaps caused by not having enough trained psychiatrists, psychologists, and social workers. Needless to say, innovative techniques of all sorts are much in evidence. Although admission rates have climbed, patient populations remain below the 1955 level, largely because the antipsychotic drugs have facilitated rapid discharge.

After discharge from the state hospital (and most patients are discharged these days), the patient's follow-up care is handled in various ways. He may be referred back to his family physician with follow-up instructions relative to his medications. Some state hospital systems operate outpatient clinics for either long-or short-term care of the previously hospitalized patient. The patient may be referred to a private psychiatrist or to the psychiatric service of a charity or university hospital. Information may or may not be forwarded to such a facility. The patient may be referred back to the community mental health center in his area for follow-up care.

Obviously, communications, or the lack of them, will be of tremendous importance to the long-term care of the patient. It is too easy for the patient to run out of his medication and fail to get more. In any event, he usually needs supervision both as to his medication and to the manner in which he deals with the normal exigencies of life. In our experience, the patient is often lost in the shuffle due to the many difficulties of communication between large systems. It behooves the physician, then, when involved in a referral process between himself and a large institutional system, to expend every effort to clarify communications, so as to render as effective medical care as possible.

Private Psychiatric Facilities

In this section, we will survey the area of the private practice of psychiatry as to its logistics, leaving its techniques to Chapter I and its referral problems to Chapter V. We will look at the private psychiatric hospital and what it may offer and the general hospital with a psychiatric division. We will conclude with a look at the private practitioner of psychiatry and examine briefly his *modus operandi*.

The Private Psychiatric Hospital: Historically, private psychiatric facilities were *spas* and *watering places* for the wealthy, taking their origin on the Continent. Treatment often consisted of hot packs, cold packs, hot baths, cold baths, bed rest, exercise, dinner parties, dances, walks in the fresh air and sunshine, massage, inspirational programs, or variations of any or all these methods. It was not uncommon for the wealthy, when life became tedious or difficult, to make their annual pilgrimage to their favorite "watering holes." Variations in diet were of the utmost importance. Surcease from anxiety and boredom was the goal. Instances of *bona fide* psychiatric illness were frequently seen, but their long-term care, in the case of hopeless mental disease, was usually left to the family who often secluded the patient on the family estate in the care of servants.

The day of the *spa* is pretty much a thing of the past; however, the revolution in psychiatric care is very apparent in the modern private psychiatric hospital. Indeed, many important advances in psychiatric theory have grown out of research and study in some of these private hospitals—Chestnut Lodge, Menninger's, The Mayo Clinic, Timberlawn, the Institute of Living. These private hospitals usually have university affiliations and are involved in research and the teaching of medical students, psychiatric residents, nursing students, aides, and other paramedical personnel.

Because the private psychiatric hospital usually has a favorable staff-patient ratio, a multifaceted approach to the patient and his problem is possible. All the treatment modalities may be available: psychopharmacology; somatic therapies; all kinds of psychotherapy —group, individual, psychoanalytic, family, couples', psychodrama; conditioning techniques; milieu therapy; and others. The patient's problems may be approached in regard to his total life situation—family, marriage, children, job. Collaboration among the various professionals over the patient's life situation frequently serves to clarify the multidetermined problems in all his life areas. In our experience, it is not at all unusual for the patient to be seen several times weekly in intensive psychotherapy, be in group therapy one to three times weekly, interact intensively in various peer group functions on his ward, undertake various classes devoted to communications and feelings, work with his wife in conjoint therapy, and engage in the various social activities of the hospital, as well as recreational and occupational therapy. While not wishing to seem to put forth a "shot-gun" approach to the patient's therapy, we are aware that the private hospital is often able to tailor a definitive treatment program for the patient, rather than attempting to fit the patient to the existing program.

Such a program, as we described in the previous paragraph, requires a tremendous amount of collaboration on the part of numerous professionals—psychiatrists, psychologists, social workers, psychiatric nurses, occupational therapists, and recreational therapists, not to mention a fair amount of hospital time for the patient. Such a treatment program is expensive; if it were not, similar programs might be more common in nonprivate facilities. Fortunately, modern health insurance plans are putting private care within the reach of more and more people, not just the wealthy. Unfortunately, federal comprehensive health care proposals seldom include provisions for psychiatric care, and what is included seems minimal to many in psychiatry. Psychiatry and its treatment modalities, are at best often cumbersome, expensive, and time-consuming; however, few substitutes or short-cuts have as yet been found, and both the patient and his psychiatrist can usually expect a lot of hard work over a prolonged period of time.

General Hospital Psychiatric Facilities: It seems beyond doubt that the majority of hospitalized psychiatric patients are currently in general hospitals. The growth of mental health services in private general hospitals is one of the well-known facts of current medical life. While formerly it was often difficult to admit a patient with a psychiatric diagnosis to a general hospital because of fears of agitated behavior, acting out potential, suicide, or homocide, it is now common to see the standard psychiatric diagnoses on admitting papers instead of fictitious diagnoses used to delude admission committees in the past.

The admissions of patients with psychiatric diagnoses may be one of the very hopeful signs in the rapprochement between psychiatrists and their fellow medical practitioners. Indeed, psychiatric consultation is available in most large city general hospitals. Many general hospitals are adding psychiatric units to their existing facilities or increasing already existing psychiatric space. New psychiatric treaments modalities are being implemented approaching the treatment milieu of the private psychiatric hospitals.

There are numerous drawbacks to incorporating psychiatric units into general hospitals—space allocation, location within traditional hospital buildings that do not provide for recreational and occupational-type therapies, limitations on the types of ancillary personnel not easily compared in the traditional medical model, continuing antipathy on the part of some members of the other specialties. However, the benefits of such an endeavor would seem to outweigh the objections—total care for the patients, opportunities of interdisciplinary study, teaching, and research, and the re-anastomosis of the "limb" of psychiatry to the "body" of medicine.

In short, the general hospital has felt the pressure of the mental health movement and has responded by increasing its psychiatric services for the benefit of the patient. We would predict this expansion to continue with the exciting possibility of full-scale mental health facilities coming into existence in most large general hospitals in the foreseeable future.

The Private Psychiatrist: There is no easy way to describe the activities of the modern psychiatrist, as he fulfills no one specific role. There is, instead, a continuum of roles that he plays. We shall attempt to look at several different types of psychiatrists as to the services they offer their patients and fellow physicians. The referring physician should be aware of these different role concepts and make every attempt to ascertain from his consultant the manner in which he conducts his practice.

The general psychiatrist is one who may conduct his daily professional life in a manner similar to a general practitioner. He will have a combined office and hospital practice. He will manage patients in the hospital with varying types of therapies—EST, insulin, groups, milieu, drugs. He will also be available to his colleagues for consultation about their patients suspected of psychological problems. His hospital practice, then, is likely to encompass a large portion of his day. His office routine is varied and busy. He has numerous patients whom he maintains on appropriate medications. He evaluates outpatients for his colleagues. He listens, counsels, advises, prescribes, sustains. If he has time and the interest, he will devote a portion of his day to more classical psychotherapy. He performs a most vital service, and he is an extremely busy man. It is almost unbelievable the phone calls that arise in the course of managing just one disturbed patient.

The psychoanalyst is a highly trained and subspecialized individual. He is, in this country, a Doctor of Medicine, a trained psychiatrist, and the graduate of a psychoanalytic institute approved by the American Psychoanalytic Association. He has spent several years undergoing his own training analysis. He frequently spends many hours per week teaching in medical schools and psychiatric residency training programs. If he practices strict psychoanalysis, he will see each patient four to five hours per week for an excess of three years. Because of the length of treatment time and his usual teaching functions, the psychoanalyst is able to see in his professional lifetime a severely restricted number of patients. His object is a thorough examination and overhaul of his patient's intrapsychic functioning. Psychoanalysis is a rigorous discipline for both patient and analyst. The analyst, except in private hospital settings, sees few hospitalized patients. Because of the rigors of analysis, the expense, the small number of trained analysts, and the limited usefulness of this procedure, few people will undergo analysis. For the ones who do successfully, the rewards are potentially great. Psychoanalysis, ultimately, is a treatment method for very few, but it is of inestimable value in teaching and research.

The role of the psychotherapist is more difficult to define. It lies somewhere between that of the general psychiatrist and the psychoanalyst. He is trained in both approaches. He may see hospitalized patients, but he sees them primarily to evaluate them for the possibility of psychotherapy. He prescribes medication, but usually he prescribes it as an adjunct to psychotherapy. He understands psychoanalytic theory and may employ psychoanalytic techniques such as the couch and free association, but he does not strive for total intrapsychic enlightenment. He will see a patient from one to five times weekly and perhaps for several years, but his interest usually lies in a segmental understanding of his patient's psychopathology. He desires to bring those intrapsychic forces obstructing the patient's adaptation to life into a closer approximation with reality and happiness. Some view this as "patch work psychoanalysis" or even "wild analysis." But in its own way, psychotherapy is a field unto itself, deserving of respect as a subspecialty of psychiatry.

The administrative psychiatrist is one who utilizes to the fullest the skills of an executive physician. He generally works in an institutional setting and is concerned with the overall management of his patients. He uses his knowledge of psychodynamics and psychiatric theory to program treatment for his patients. He is the contact between his patient and the patient's family. If the patient is "in therapy" with another psychiatrist, he is the mediator between the fantasy of the couch and the reality of the world. All in all, his importance is extreme but, unfortunately, frequently underrated. His skills are special and highly varied. He prescribes various psychotropic drugs and must be proficient in their usages. He often testifies at commitment and child custody hearings as an expert witness. He conducts ward management practices of the utmost subtlety and sophistication. He is responsible for the operation of the milieu program of his ward. He is legally responsible for all that happens to his patients on a daily basis. He must select the other highly specialized treatment techniques that might benefit his patients. He must stay in contact with the referring physician and apprise him of the direction and results of treatment with each individual patient. At the same time, many administrative psychiatrists are accomplished psychotherapists, although most choose to work with patients for whom they are not administratively responsible. All in all, the administrative psychiatrist, within the profession, is one of the most highly regarded of all psychiatrists.

The foregoing synopses can only serve to skim the surface of the various functions of the private psychiatrist. Many private psychiatrists devote much of their time *gratis* to teaching. Others, with interests in legal medicine, consult with various governmental agencies. Some work in community mental health centers part-time, at V.A. outpatient clinics, or donate their time to other community endeavors. What we are describing, then, are specialties within a specialty, difficult of definition but important as to functions.

Parapsychiatric Facilities

In addition to the described medical referral facilities, the referring physician has at his disposal numerous nonmedical facilities to which he may refer his patient. These facilities and professionals are more difficult to categorize broadly, but a general summary is offered as being reasonably complete.

The Psychologist: The functions of the psychologist are particularly hard to categorize. He usually is a Ph.D., although he may in some areas of the country be an Ed.D. Training varies widely. Some psychologists have no clinical orientation and, thus, are excluded from our consideration. Many clinical psychologists are interested in psychological testing procedures and are extremely useful to the psychiatric evaluation as the psychiatrist is seldom adept in these testing procedures. Testing procedures are varied and multitudinous—intellectual functioning, personality inventory, job preference scales, depressive scales, tests for cerebral organicity, and projective techniques. It is beyond the scope of this monograph to pursue the topic of testing further; therefore, the student is referred to a standard reference on such testing procedures.

A psychologist may devote his time to the various social agencies of the community. He may teach in a university or medical school. He may consult in school systems. He may be in private practice and receive patients much as does a physician. He often performs psychotherapy, either group, individual, or family. He may specialize in adult or adolescent and child psychology. He may or may not be licensed or certified by the state in which he practices.

The Social Worker: The duties and functions of the social worker are, as with the psychologist, difficult to categorize broadly. He, or more commonly she, although more and more men are entering the field, usually has an M.S.W. Degree (Master of Social Work) or an M.S.S.W. Degree (Master of Science in Social Work). The more experienced workers will be accredited by the American College of Social Workers and bear the title ACSW after their names. The protean duties of the social worker include working for social agencies in many areas of human deprivation, teaching in college and medical schools, working in psychiatric clinics and hospitals, consulting in school systems, and some are currently in private practice. Although most do not engage in traditional psychotherapy, many are extremely adept at the various forms of counselling procedures, marital, job, child care, family, and group. Because of their skills in investigating and working with family and social processes, the social worker is usually an integral part of the mental health team.

The Psychiatric Nurse: All members of the mental health team have become more highly specialized. This is true, also, of the psychiatric nurse. Of recent origin are degree programs designed to award the Masters and Ph.D. degrees in psychiatric nursing. Few psychiatric nurses are as yet in private practice, but their place in aiding the team approach to improving mental health functioning is unique and important.

Miscellaneous Resources: In this section, we are lumping together a group of resources of varied nature to give the physician an overview of the numerous facilities available. The grouping by no means covers the field, nor is it intended to. Neither have we chosen to deal with the issue of the charlatan or untrained "counsellor." As we have tangentially noted, one often does not have to be licensed or certified to engage in counseling. Indeed, in many areas of the country, one only has to declare himself a counsellor in order to receive payment for his services. The physician is encouraged to examine carefully the credentials and references of the consultant or counsellor to which he is considering referring his patient.

Ministerial counselling is of extremely ancient origin, taking its roots both from religion and primitive medicine. He is the evolutionary offspring of the witch doctor, shaman, obeah man, and priest. The minister is constantly under pressure by his parishioners to help deal with their numerous problems. Until recently, he usually relied on common sense, intuition, and prayer to deal with these numerous problems. Of late, divinity schools and seminaries have become more interested in counselling procedures and mental health problems. The minister is receiving a more thorough grounding in psychology, sociology, and psychoanalytic theory. Because of their increasing interest in this field, a new breed of helper, the ministerial counsellor has evolved. In the large church, his sole job is counselling with the troubled of the parish, while the preaching is left to his counterpart. Since there is no standard method of accrediting such counsellors, the referring physician is encouraged to use his own powers of observation in determining the skill and usefulness of such an individual practitioner.

The psychiatric volunteer is a relatively new entity in medicine and often viewed with suspicion by nonpsychiatric medical people.[7]

Because of the paucity of trained personnel, the psychiatrist has sometimes turned to bright, dedicated, interested, trainable lay people to assist him in performing certain duties in the psychiatric clinic, such as administering psychological tests, taking developmental histories, assisting in intake groups, and performing other responsibilities usually reserved for more highly trained personnel. These people are always closely supervised by professional members of the psychiatric team, and can be useful adjuncts in the health care delivery efforts of the team.

Varying techniques, philosophies, and approaches are encountered when surveying the numerous alcoholic treatment centers in this country; they may or may not be of psychiatric orientation and influence. They may or may not be operated by physicians. At last report, there were in excess of 9 million alcoholics in the United States, and treatment and rehabilitation programs have not been uniformly beneficial.

Social Agencies: A description of the kinds and activities of social agencies in our modern society would require a large volume unto itself. Social concerns, increasing through years of education, affluence, and mass transportation and communications, have required all branches of governments, local, state, and federal, to take an increasing interest in the well-being of our society's citizens. At present, almost all levels of society are involved with one or more social agencies—child welfare, adoptions, veterans' problems, aid to the dependent and ill, Social Security, the blind, lame, and halt, widows and orphans, criminals and delinquents, economically advantaged and economically deprived. Involved in each of these agencies are social workers, psychologists, and psychiatrists. The full weight of the law and court opinion lies behind their endeavors. It is confusing and virtually impossible for the busy physician to acquire a full understanding of all these varied and overlapping functions, yet he daily comes into contact with them, often without being aware of the contact. Even the psychiatrist, who is often highly involved with social agencies, has difficulty sorting out the material regarding the areas of responsibility for the various agencies. Social workers are generally more cognizant of the intricacies of this referral process. Many large cities have central information centers, such as the Council of Social Agencies, which are able to disseminate the necessary information to the referring physician. The increase in the complexity of this referral process is likely to parallel the increase in the general complexity of our society.

Child and Adolescent Services

The mental health of children and adolescents is receiving increasing scrutiny, the impetus coming from increases in juvenile delinquency rates and drug-related problems. The President's Commission on the Mental Health of Children has added fuel to the fire by bringing public attention to the sad plight of many children in this country. Child and adolescent treatment facilities are increasing, but the unhappy fact is that there are by no means enough facilities in this country even to evaluate these young people, much less treat them.

The child guidance movement in this country is many years old and has done fine service in helping children and training child psychiatrists. There are, however, relatively few child psychiatrists and psychologists in the United States. Child guidance clinics are found only in the larger cities and have long waiting lists.

The field of adolescent psychiatry is new, and has jointly been approached in a cooperative way by both child and adult psychiatrists, for it is generally agreed that adolescence cannot be the exclusive domain of either group. The American Society for Adolescent Psychiatry and the Pan-American Federation of Societies for Adolescent Psychiatry have agreed jointly that special techniques for treating adolescents are mandatory. They have been encouraging psychiatric residency training programs to teach these methods, and a whole new body of literature relating to this stormy period of life is developing.

In the meantime, adolescent services and programs are being organized at juvenile departments, general and university hospitals, state hospitals, and private hospitals. Special private schools for emotionally disturbed children and adolescents are hard at work. Unfortunately, the hospitalization of an adolescent is usually lengthy, expensive, and not assured of success. Special camps, both summer and year-round, have been organized to attempt a different approach to adolescent treatment programs.[8]

The problems of childhood and adolescence are receiving increasing emphasis, but the ultimate answer is likely to be a long way off. The referring physician will need to seek guidance in this area from school and juvenile authorities, psychiatrists and social agencies when he is faced with referring the child or adolescent.

Summary

We make no apologies for the foregoing discussion of the consulting facilities available to the referring physician when determining the direction of a psychiatric referral. The complexity is a product of our society. We do feel the physician should have at least an overview of this area, as there is no way he can escape involvement with it sooner or later. It does illustrate rather graphically that the referral process is difficult, and the physician should be aware that the psychiatrist has to grapple daily with this particularly confusing and complicated problem. The physician, by now, is also aware that the psychiatrist must, of necessity, relate regularly with many or all these governmental organizations and agencies in an effort to aid the psychiatric patient.

Chapter IV

TECHNIQUES OF
REFERRAL

P ATIENT ACCEPTANCE OF PSYCHIATRY varies considerably among different parts of the country and also among social classes. The eastern portion of the country tolerated psychiatry first, and indeed, in certain areas, having one's "own" psychiatrist or analyst has become a mark of distinction and an indication of high social status. Conversely, acceptance of psychiatry has only lately begun to appear in the South and Midwest. Curiously, it appears that the highest and the lowest socioeconomic classes in all parts of the country have the most contact with and understanding and acceptance of the role of the psychiatrist in modern medical practice. The juxtaposition of these two diverse classes' acceptance has come about due to widely divergent causes, namely affluence and education in the higher class and influence of the Community Mental Health Centers in the lower.

The large numbers of persons comprising the middle class, which of course makes up the bulk of the private physician's practice, have, until recently, escaped the full impact of our society's acceptance of psychiatry. The physician, who generally is a member of the middle class, also is representative of the lack of contact with and suspiciousness toward psychiatry and the psychiatrist.

In this monograph we are concerned only with the patient who is referred by his physician to a psychiatrist and not the person who, on his own recognizance, seeks such help himself without utilization of the referral process. The referral process, then, being a study in interpersonal relations between nonpsychiatric physicians and psychiatrists, is open to inspection from the standpoints of both the referrent and the consultant—not as a means of meting out criticism, nor to attack or blame one or the other, but to attempt to let a little light fall on a most difficult area. This chapter, then, will approach the referral problem from the viewpoint of the nonpsychiatric physician.

Language Problem: Harry Stack Sullivan once criticized psychiatry for its development of a separate and unnecessarily complicated language. (He then proceeded, in effect, to develop another, and perhaps even more complicated language.) The language barrier between psychiatrists and referrents is imposing, and indeed, psychiatrists do not necessarily understand one another well if trained in different schools of psychiatric thought. At the beginning of the therapeutic relationship, then, there exists a strangeness in communication. This strangeness often results in suspiciousness and hostility. What one does not understand, one usually does not trust. The physician's lack of trust and confidence in psychiatry is easily betrayed to the patient he is referring. Some have attributed this attitude to lack of sophistication about psychological ideas or to the general physician's own problems and his unconscious use of his defense mechanisms in dealing with his own anxiety and anger toward psychiatry. Undoubtedly, this does occur, but it would seem also that the profound language barrier that exists may be equally, if not more, important. Hopefully, this barrier may become more inconsequential as medical schools across the country adopt more sophisticated approaches to psychological medicine. Indeed, considering that psychiatry only became a major recognized portion of the medical school curriculum following World War II, much improvement is already seen. Certainly it is the responsibility of the medical schools to ensure in the future the proper exposure of the medical student to a reasonably thorough understanding of psychological medicine and its terminology.

Physician Attitudes: Without wishing to offend, but at the same time recognizing, that, if the referral process is to undergo improvement, we will need to examine objectively the nonpsychiatric physician's attitudes toward psychiatry. In the next chapter, we will perform the same objective service for the psychiatric consultant. Perhaps, since one of us has spent a good many years in general practice, internal medicine, and psychiatry, this objectivity will be more real than apparent.

There is no question but that the manner in which the nonpsychiatric physician refers his patient to a psychiatrist is influenced by his own unconscious conflicts along with society's fear of insanity. The physician may view a neurosis through his own fears of his possible neurotic makeup. He may see a marital conflict through the distortions of his own marriage. Certainly, religious and political beliefs are a fertile ground for censorship of the patient and his conflicts as well as the psychiatrist. The physician, then, may be suspicious of psychiatry due to his suspiciousness of his own unconscious psychical forces, and project this same suspiciousness onto the psychiatrist. In the meantime, he transmits this suspiciousness to his patient in an antitherapeutic manner. It goes without saying that the success of the contact between psychiatrist and patient is often predicated upon the referring physician's tact and the skillful manner in which he makes the referral. To emphasize once again, we feel that the manner in which the medical school deals with the student physician's feelings about psychiatry and his own intrapsychic makeup will be of paramount importance in the referral process and the care of the patient with psychological problems. The physician who finds that his hostility and apprehension toward psychiatry are interfering with his ability to assist the patient who consults him for psychological problems will, perhaps, desire to discuss this area with someone trained to help him relieve his anxiety.

The physician may have trained in a time before many of the advances in psychological medicine were made, and he may be unaware of the numerous patients psychiatry is now able to help. It may be difficult for others to differentiate the successes in psychiatric intervention from the numerous psychiatric treatment failures. The thoughtful physician will want to reflect on the proposition that there are malignant psychiatric disorders just as there are malignant tumors. The sociopathies, alcohol and drug addictions, and the perversions are examples where psychiatry has not enjoyed particular success.

At the same time, it is apparent that psychiatry has "oversold" itself. The mass media extoll the fruits of mental health intervention. The physician often expects too much from the psychiatrist and is disappointed at the lack of results. As we have mentioned in an earlier chapter, the former view that the psychosomatic disorders could be effectively treated by psychotherapy has drastically changed. Thus, the asthmatic, the ulcer patient, the hypertensive patient, the arthritic are thrust back upon the physician for care after the proud pronouncements that these illnesses have combined somatic and psychical causes.

Treatment failures occur in all areas of psychiatry as in all other branches of medicine. The neurosis may fail to respond after long and expensive psychotherapy or psychoanalysis. The patient with somatic symptoms may, in fact, be dealing with such tremendous personal, psychological, and social problems that he finds psychiatry poorly equipped to help him. The apparently successfully treated psychosis may return, to the consternation of both patient and physician.

Psychiatry, of all the medical sciences, is the least exact and scientific. It is not antiscientific, but because of its relationship to the social sciences and its necessary reliance on verbal data, thoughts, fantasies, and dreams, it becomes more of an art, in many respects, than a science. On the other hand, it has become more scientific, and likely it will become even more so, but its position of acting as a bridge between medicine and the social sciences will and should remain. It deals with abstractions. Psychiatrists think in psychodynamic terminology and discuss what cannot be seen and, indeed, does not exist—ego, id, superego. Medical schools, in general, must be cited for their tendencies to encourage student physicians to think in concrete terms and be suspicious of what they cannot see.

Common Referral Errors: While not desiring to encompass an encyclopedic approach and list all possible errors of referral, it does seem appropriate, at the same time, to delve into some of the more common errors that make for a great deal of difficulty in the referral process.

Misinforming the Patient: Because of shyness, anxiety, lack of understanding, or feelings about his own inability to diagnose or treat the patient, the physician frequently, consciously or unconsciously, undermines the psychiatrist-patient relationship before it begins by transmitting faulty or distorted information to the patient. The physician may refer to the psychiatrist as a "nerve specialist," thus implying that the patient will see a neurologist or neurosurgeon. This appellation suggests there is something wrong with the patient's central nervous system, nerves, brain, spine, etc. It, most unfortunately of all, denies the possible existence of psychological processes at work which have caused the patient's discomfort. It reaffirms the *soma* at the expense of the *psyche* as the area for investigation. It will almost always cause embarrassment to both patient and psychiatrist when the "truth" comes out; the consultant is a psychiatrist and not a "nerve specialist." Great anger can be anticipated on the part of both psychiatrist and patient because the patient, has, in effect, been lied to.

Another unfortunate, but by no means uncommon, deception is not to tell the patient at all that he will be seen by a psychiatrist. One who has not been in this position cannot understand the anger and humiliation felt by both psychiatrist and patient. That little can be expected from the interview is an understatement. The physician referring in these circumstances may well expect little information forthcoming from the consultation, which is likely to further his own antipathy toward psychiatry. The subtle message to the patient is that he would have objected to being seen by a psychiatrist and thus was deceived. The message to the consultant is that he and his specialty are repugnant to the referring physician, and thus to be denied and avoided as much as possible.

It is not unheard of for the physician with this view of psychiatry to use a referral to "scare" the patient into getting better; the "threat" of the psychiatrist is thus utilized to reproach the patient for having only psychical problems, therefore shameful and not deserving of respect as would be accorded a more respectable somatic illness. This "boogey man" approach will usually turn the patient against both the psychiatrist and the referring physician, which may also be the desired effect of the referral. Unfortunately, this is not the recommended way for a physician to rid himself of an "undesirable" patient whose symptoms the physician is no longer able to tolerate. Also, the psychiatrist will usually resent being the instrument of the patient's separation from his physician.

Instead, the physician should clearly and without apology (for none is needed) inform his patient that he desires an investigation into the possible psychological causes of the patient's illness or discomfort. He should clearly inform the patient he will be seen by Dr. X, a psychiatrist, for purposes of this investigation. This knowledge should be transmitted as understandingly and matter-of-factly as if the patient were being referred to another type of specialist. If one treats his patient as a competent adult, usually the patient, despite his psychological regression due to illness and discomfort, will respond as a responsible adult. He has the right to understand clearly the significance of his referral, and he can better utilize the help of the consultant by being prepared to cooperate with the consultant toward his own improvement. Psychiatry is, after all, one of many medical specialties, and it is best for the patient and the consultation that it be approached in that light. Psychiatrists, as well as all other physicians, are seekers after the truth; therefore, it is seldom helpful when looking for the truth to begin with lies, distortions, omissions, or deceptions.

Failing to Refer: If the physician denies psychiatry's importance as a useful medical specialty, then he may also deny his patient the opportunity for help he often painfully requires. The physician's denial, albeit unconscious, may enable him to miss many important diagnostic clues of anxiety, depression, imminent suicide. The most common oversight relates to the patient whose numerous somatic complaints mask a depression. The physician, in this instance, treats the symptoms instead of the illness, and leaves the patient to suffer, while the physician becomes more uncomfortable with his own inability to relieve the patient's suffering. He may eventually, due to his own anxiety, dismiss the patient as a "crock" or a "hypochondriac," never appreciating that he is treating a severely depressed human being. While delving into the "hypochondriac's" numerous somatic symptoms, the physician should ever be alert to the possibility that a depression lurks beneath the ubiquitous bodily complaints, and it behooves him to inquire tactfully of the patient's emotional situation as well. Surprisingly, the patient is usually ready to voice his latent feelings of depression, worthlessness, impotence, deficiency of self-esteem, concerns about his marriage or children or parents, suicidal ruminations, anxieties, fears, phobias, or loss of self-respect. The patient may, on the other hand, be surprised that anyone is interested in his psychological feelings, because he is usually the person who finds a deaf ear when he voices his feelings, and he unconsciously turns to somatic symptoms that enable him to find someone, family or physician, who will feel it acceptable to listen to him. The physician may also develop the skill of inquiring into his patient's feelings about his own death, and he may be surprised at the relief the patient experiences in tearfully telling how he wishes he were dead. The physician should not be fearful of discussing suicide, as such a discussion often turns the impulse into words instead of into the dreaded action. Once these feelings are out in the open, both doctor and patient can decide what appropriate measures should be undertaken for the patient's relief, and of course, the psychiatric referral may then be approached in a more cooperative and helpful way. Patients are almost always grateful when their physicians evince understanding of their psychological as well as their somatic feelings.

Ruling Out Organic Illness: The busy physician frequently is unable to separate out the physical complaints of his patient regarding *psyche vs. soma,* and we frequently hear the physician say: "I wish I knew a psychiatrist I could send a patient to and find out if the patient is suffering from a psychological illness." We hear great bitterness in his spoken wish, and we understand the dilemma that he faces; however, unfortunate as it is, although a psychiatrist may be highly skilled in interview techniques, there is no substitute for the physician's thorough physical and laboratory examination. Depressions often mask organic illnesses such as carcinoma and brain tumor. The organic brain syndrome may be due to brain tumor. Anxiety may be due to physical causes of which the patient hesitates to admit or of which he is only vaguely aware. The psychiatrist, then, has the right to expect of the referring physician that he has thoroughly examined the patient, and to the best of his ability, has ruled out organic sources for the patient's discontent. The reverse, at present, cannot be true, since the psychiatrist has few testing tools at his disposal to separate somatic from psychical complaints. The report of his examination should be made known to the psychiatrist at the time of the psychiatric evaluation.

The Late or Last Minute Referral: As we discussed in Chapter I, some hospitals make it a practice to require that all patients admitted for suicidal attempts or gestures be examined by the psychiatric consultant prior to discharge. The numerous objections to this have been voiced in Chapter I. Suffice it to say that the psychiatric consultant functions best as a member of the medical team rather than as one who assumes legal or moral responsibility as to whether the patient will or will not harm someone.

In the same vein, the physician often requires a psychiatric consultation just prior to the patient's discharge. Sometimes he implies: "We don't want to leave out any diagnostic procedure, no matter how slight the chance of success." At other times he may want to clear himself legally and professionally by passing the responsibility to an "authority." It may also be a reflection of the physician's idea of his role as one who only rules out organic disease. Unfortunately, the last minute consultation implies the psychiatric evaluation is of little importance. It, in effect, denigrates the importance of the patient's psychological life and problems, and sets the stage for further denial by the physician and his patient. This sort of consultation is almost always a failure. The artificiality, either overt or implied, of the separation between *psyche* and *soma* further intensifies the problems of the patient who is having trouble understanding that his bodily symptoms may be of psychological origin.

The psychiatric referral, then, should be made when other tests and consultations are ordered so that the patient will understand his total bodily and psychological functions are being investigated in a unitarian approach. The physician shows his patient his acceptance of the importance of the patient's emotional functions and helps his patient accept those functions as normal and respectable. The psychiatrist has the opportunity to establish professional rapport with the patient in the event that psychiatric intervention becomes a necessity. This approach also allows the psychiatrist the opportunity of being involved in the team decision-making on behalf of the patient prior to surgery or acute psychiatric disturbance.

Surgical Persuasion: Two authors, Weiner[16] and Liddon[10], have taken umbrage at "the last-minute consultation before surgery." In the cases they cite, the consultation is undertaken just prior to scheduled surgery, in which event the psychiatrist is expected to "sell" the surgery, and is viewed by the patient as an obstacle to the desired procedure rather than a member of the health care delivery team. Failure on the part of the psychiatrist may be expected as he is usually not trained in sales techniques.

Referral Suggestions:

Up to this point, we have tried to describe some problem areas related to: what to refer, when to refer, whom to refer, where to refer, and, hopefully, how not to refer. It is always the easier task to be critical, dogmatic, and condemnatory, which is not at all the purpose of this monograph, although some criticism of both referring physician and consultant is not to be avoided if honesty, which should be the hallmark of medicine, is not to be circumvented. We prefer to see this endeavor as a positive approach to the interpersonal relationship between physician and psychiatrist with the patient's best interests the common goal. Therefore, we would like to offer these tentative suggestions for the physician's happier and smoother relationship with his psychiatrist colleague. The thoughtful practitioner will add numerous other suggestions out of the depth of his experience in this shadowy area. He is encouraged to do so, for our purpose, hopefully, is to stimulate further thought, rather than to promulgate dogma in an area already too complicated by dogma and prejudice. Pragmatism is, in most instances, superior to dogmatism, and certainly a pragmatic approach to helping the patient is the physician's desired professional function. Then, these suggestions are to be taken as what they represent—suggestions only.

Knowing the Consultant: It may seem trite to emphasize such an obvious point, but realistically, interpersonal relationships are best engaged in between people who know each other at least fairly well. The unfortunate point is that many physicians only superficially know their psychiatric consultants, if at all. We will look at the psychiatrist's part in this in the next chapter. Suffice it to say for now that most physicians know fairly well their other consultants: ENT, surgery, ob-gyn, etc. A certain distance exists between the referring physician and his psychiatric consultant, and this interpersonal gap serves to further complicate the referral process. The reasons for this gap have and will be discussed further, but it will serve the physician's purpose well if he will acquire a reasonable knowledge of his psychiatric consultant and/or facility. He should know what he can reasonably expect from his consultant. The relationship preferably should exist prior to the need for a specific referral. He should know generally what the consultant is prepared to do for the patient and the area of psychiatry at which he is most adept. Clarity of communication is essential.

The physician's reasons for referring will vary from patient to patient, and he clearly needs to state what he wants each time even if he routinely deals with a single psychiatric consultant. One time he may want only an evaluation. Another time he may want both evaluation and an outline of a treatment program which he can then implement himself. Still another time he may want the consultant not only to provide the evaluation, but also to conduct any indicated treatment or make arrangements for it. We have not cited the situation in which a patient is referred for treatment only, and a word ought to be said about that. Hopefully, a referring physician does not do this; presumably the first step in the service of any consultant is to make an evaluation of the referral situation. To tell a patient he is being referred for ECT or hospitalization or lithium, for example, is placing the consultant in the potentially awkward position of disagreeing with the referring doctor's assessment of the patient.

The Somatic Examination: The physician, as has been stated in a previous section, should be prepared to furnish the psychiatrist a detailed work-up, verbal or written, of the patient's general physical condition along with the usual and necessary laboratory and Xray determinations. When the patient is referred to the consultant, the physician often will find it necessary to maintain his professional concern for the patient's physical condition as the psychiatrist cannot replace this function in most instances of outpatient care. (This does not apply to university hospitals, V.A. hospitals, state psychiatric hospitals, or private psychiatric hospitals.) Often, because the physician has maintained total care for his patient, both somatic and emotional, he may find it difficult, due to his normal feelings of omnipotence, to give up his prerogatives in relation to the patient's psychological care. While he should be as completely informed as possible regarding what the psychiatrist is doing for his patient—psychotherapy, ECT, psychotropic drugs—he will find it more appropriate to reserve his remarks and feelings about such treatment for the psychiatrist's ear so as not to encourage doubt in the patient about his psychiatric care. Particularly while in psychotherapy, the patient will mobilize all sorts of extraneous negative opinions into the service of his unconscious resistances to therapy. If the physician is able to be supportive of the psychiatrist in a positive way, without being judgmental, interpretive, or obstructive, the patient stands a better chance to improve. If the physician has doubts, he should convey them to the psychiatrist for discussion. After all, the physician chose the consultant, and it would be inappropriate to undermine the very treatment he instigated. Often, the patient will unknowingly provoke the physician to pass judgment on the treatment he is receiving. Again, this is usually in the service of unconscious resistances on the patient's part.

Frankness with the Patient: At all times, frankness, honesty, and truthfulness are appropriate when the physician is referring his patient to a psychiatric consultant. Deception is never appropriate. On the other hand, this does not demand that the physician reveal his unproved concerns, suspicions, or doubts about the patient's condition. He should honestly tell the patient he feels the patient's symptoms, which have not been proved to be of organic cause, may be of emotional origin. A common mistake is to imply these symptoms are imaginary or "in the head." To the patient, the symptoms are real and as deserving of respect, tolerance, and acceptance on the part of the physician as any physical pain known. Indeed, few patients commit suicide because of the pain of childbirth or renal calculi.

At the same time, the physician will not want to hide his real concern. A genuine awareness of this concern is often reassuring to the patient that the physician cares about him and is seeking to alleviate his suffering by the referral. It is never appropriate to make light of the patient's referral as this subserves the function of increasing the patient's denial. Acknowledging suffering is always more comforting than pretending it will go away.

The patient may be embarrassed at referral to a psychiatrist. It may, to him, represent moral weakness or mental laxity. Insanity is much feared. His embarrassment should be acknowledged, but the physician may find it useful to put the psychiatric referral in the same light as referral to any other medical specialist, thus recognizing the importance of the patient's emotional life but not attaching undue emphasis to the emotional over the somatic functions. If the patient is told that the psychiatric consultant is a Doctor of Medicine especially trained in understanding the patient's mental processes and emotional life, he generally will be more accepting of the referral.

To reiterate, the patient should be told that his physician feels the patient's problems and symptoms may be of emotional or psychological origin, and that in order to investigate such a possibility, he is referring the patient to a psychiatrist, who is a Doctor of Medicine specializing in emotional factors. It is helpful, also, if the physician can reflect to the patient some confidence in the psychiatrist's competence in his profession. Ideally, the timing should be such that the consultant has the opportunity to make a thorough evaluation and advise with the patient and his physician as to his suggestions for further care. The foregoing should be approached with all the professional skill and concern that the physician utilizes in his everyday professional life. The skill and care, concern and competence, with which the physician refers his patient for psychiatric care will, in large measure, determine the final outcome of his patient's disorder and the rapidity with which he returns to his normal activities.

Chapter V

WHAT TO EXPECT
FROM THE CONSULTANT

T HE AIM OF THIS CHAPTER is to implement the physician's efforts
to get what he needs from a psychiatric referral by better acquaint-
ing him with what it is that psychiatrists have to offer. Here we are
talking not about specific treatment facilities or treatment modalities (topics already discussed in Chapters II and III), but rather
about basic approaches to patients and to other doctors—in other
words, the particular skills that psychiatrists as professionals have
to offer their patients and their colleagues in other fields of medicine.

As stated in the preface, doctors as a group seem to complain
more about psychiatric referral results than they do about the
services of any other specialty. And we propose that this is because
the capabilities (and limitations) of psychiatry are rather poorly
understood by the majority of nonpsychiatrists, generalists and specialists alike.

That one field of medicine should be so susceptible to mis-
understandings by other doctors bears some looking at. The easy
explanation, and the one often given, is that no one enjoys being
reminded of his own vulnerability to emotional hang-ups. And
somehow the very existence of psychiatry as a specialty serves to
acknowledge this particular aspect of the human condition.

Another explanation, and one which we think carries greater

weight, has to do with the conflict engendered in physicians by the nature of the psychiatrist's particular tools of his trade—namely, that he proposes to help his patients by listening to them and talking with them. Now, all doctors talk and listen to their patients to greater or lesser degrees. So what are the implications of having some doctors say that this is their primary skill? Bergen and his coworkers[2] at Dartmouth talked with a number of community physicians and decided that the implications were great indeed. Underlying the community physicians' complaints about their difficulties in dealing with psychiatrists seemed to be a feeling that to ask for help with their emotionally troubled patients meant, not that they needed to refer a problem that was "out of their line," but rather that they had been less effective than the consultant was likely to be in employing a mutually held skill.

We would add that there is a flip side to this feeling. And it is the side that is more openly expressed, at least, by nonpsychiatrists. It is the feeling that psychiatrists get paid a lot for doing very little; all they do is listen to their patients, something that every good doctor throws in "for free" while attending to the real problems, the broken leg or the perforated ulcer. No one ought be challenging the fact that in terms of sheer numbers of patients, far more psychiatric problems are being handled—and often effectively—by nonpsychiatric physicians than by those with psychiatric training. But for emotional problems that are not readily resolved by the nonpsychiatrist's intervention, the psychiatrist can bring to bear a talking-listening procedure that is different from—not better than—the kind of talking-listening relationship the nonpsychiatrist effects with his patients while he is doing something else for them (be it providing prenatal care, giving their children summer camp physicals, prescribing iron pills for their anemia, or removing their mother-in-law's appendix).

The conflict seems to arise out of the confusion regarding what it is that psychiatrists do. If they only do for sizeable fees what other doctors do "for free," then they are charlatans or frauds to be viewed with contempt. If on the other hand they do with consummate skill what other doctors can only falteringly imitate, then they are a constant reproach to their medical colleagues who can only view them with awe and discomfort. Neither of these viewpoints is accurate or useful, but both, we suggest, are prevalent. And both stem from a failure to understand that the kind of listening and talking that a psychiatrist does and the very particular kind of relationship that he establishes with his patients is different from the kind of listening and talking that other physicians do. The latter works well with the majority of patients who are experiencing transient problems in living. But it is no discredit to physicians to recognize that different disorders require different treatments and that the psychiatrist, by virtue of having some different skills, not better skills, is able to treat effectively certain types of patients that do not respond to the skills of nonpsychiatrists. In Chapter I we listed these different types of patients.

Another determinant of the awe-contempt response that psychiatry seems to elicit may lie somewhere in the history of medicine. Back in medicine's primitive past physicians had their beginnings. All spring from a common source, the witch doctor or priest healer. But in modern medicine it is psychiatrists alone who serve as reminders of that humbling heritage. Physicians, if they look backward at all, recite the Hippocratic oath, not some witch doctor's chant. Thus they willingly claim Greek rationalism-naturalism as their own but leave the art of "headshrinking" to the primitives and to the psychiatrists. The widespread use of that epithet clearly conveys the mixed response of awe and contempt about which we are speaking. On the one hand "headshrinking" suggests a practice that has no scientific basis or utility while on the other hand it hints of powers that transcend science.

To the extent that psychiatry and those who practice it are seen as both superior to and inferior to all the rest of medicine, but never quite on a par with it, other physicians are destined to be disappointed with their referral results. They will be disappointed because they will either be expecting far too much or they will be expecting nothing at all. If they expect truly magical cures from healers whose skills far exceed their own, then they will refer patients who would indeed require magic to make them well. If they expect only a sort of mumbo-jumbo ritual signifying nothing and producing even less but costing a great deal more than what they themselves are fully trained to provide, then they will refer patients that they want to punish, frighten, or get rid of, but certainly not to help. In either case, for such physicians, the psychiatrist is a specialist without a useful specialty.

Every once in awhile somebody suggests that psychiatrists could get along better with other doctors and thus be of more service if they started to act more like other doctors. Proposals are made that they retrieve their stethoscopes, put on their white coats and talk about their patients the way other doctors do. Such a reversion might well increase their rapport with their colleagues but it might diminish the value of their specialty. Psychiatrists are different. They practice a different kind of medicine. And therein lies their utility.

Right from the beginning of their residency program, young psychiatrists begin learning new procedures that are notably different from those learned in any other specialty. But it is not these new procedures in themselves that set psychiatrists apart from other practitioners. After all, every specialty has its own particular techniques. What further separates them from other doctors is the unlearning that they do. They have to unlearn, in significant ways, much of what they have already been taught—medical attitudes, beliefs, and procedures that all other physicians continue to employ.

To begin with, and perhaps most importantly, they have to give up the action-oriented framework of medicine, a framework which classically sees the physician as the person who decides what is wrong with a patient, determines what to do about it, and then does it, enlisting the patient's participation only to ensure the proper following of the doctor's orders. Psychiatrists must learn to be more passive. They must content themselves with the role of facilitator, giving to the patient the tasks and satisfactions of finding out what is wrong, deciding what to do about it, and then choosing whether or not to do it.

Adding to the stress of developing this new orientation at the expense of abandoning an old, widely accepted one, is the uneasiness created by the vagueness of psychodynamics and psychopathology as compared to the more concrete world of organ physiology and pathology. Budding psychiatrists are expected to change their whole professional role and, as a rationale for the change, are offered concepts that cannot be demonstrated directly by any of the senses and that to this day remain open to challenge and to attack. The fact that the treatment methods developed out of these concepts sometimes work (and sometimes do not!) provides little comfort for the positivistic young physician. More, perhaps, than any other kind of doctor, the psychiatrist must learn to be comfortable with ambiguity and downright uncertainty if he is to survive at all. If he is to help his patients, he must then go one step further and find in these very qualities of ambiguity and uncertainty the opportunities for emotional growth that they contain. This process may well be one of the factors operative in the decision that so many psychiatric residents make to undergo psychotherapy during the course of their training.

Uncertainty troubles the neophyte psychiatrist, not just in regard to the relative vagaries of psychodynamics and psychopathology and not just in regard to being asked to abandon a medical position of authority and action. Uncertainty troubles him badly in regard to the question of who he is, professionally speaking. Not only is he unlearning ways of being like other doctors. He is, and this may be the most painful part of all, learning methods and procedures that make him appear more like certain nondoctors. The large numbers and various types of nonmedical persons offering help to the emotionally troubled can be very confusing and, at times, distressing to the young psychiatrist trying to figure out who he is and what he is supposed to be doing. (It can also be confusing and therefore distressing to the patient wanting psychiatric help and to the nonpsychiatric physician trying to facilitate the patient's search for help.) Psychologists, social workers, and clergymen form only a very partial list of non-MD's who deal in psychotherapy (see Chapter III). The last mentioned on this list see far more persons with emotional problems than do psychiatrists, and they refer on to psychiatrists only a very small fraction of those whom they see. The first two on the list, psychologists and social workers, are actually found very frequently on the teaching staffs of psychiatric training programs, not to provide ancillary services for the physicians, but to teach them how to do psychotherapy. Such an arrangement can be highly unsettling to any physician, and it has no counterpart that we know of in any other type of specialty training.

There is a term being tossed around, though not lightly, in psychiatric educational circles. The term is "identity crisis," and, in using it, medical educators are acknowledging that the stresses we have been describing above do occur and take their toll among young psychiatrists in training.[15] The question being raised and not yet adequately answered is, How can one go through the process of learning to become a psychiatrist without also going through the experience of feeling so isolated and alienated from other kinds of doctors and hence feeling so uncertain and uncomfortable with one's professional role? (Perhaps that is the wrong question and a more fruitful one would address itself not to how to avoid the identity crisis, but how to use it as a paradigm for psychotherapy. However, that would be an issue for a separate monograph.)

It may be that for most psychiatrists, at least those engaged primarily in psychotherapy, the identity crisis conflicts are not ever completely resolved; certainly, the issues of isolation and alienation seem to be major obstacles contributing to the referral dissatisfactions so many nonpsychiatrists experience in dealing with their psychiatric colleagues.

In our own experience, and judging from a small scattering of articles appearing in the psychiatric journals[13,15], referring physicians do not complain about the treatment their patients receive from psychiatrists; rather these doctors complain about the treatment that they as referring physicians receive. And what they complain about is that they are ignored. It is a remarkable paradox that the one group of medical specialists who place supreme premium upon adequate doctor-patient communication should be so seemingly remiss in their communications with other doctors. In what remains of this chapter we shall discuss what we see as the explanations for this phenomenon and consider what can be done to remedy it.

Whenever a doctor makes a referral, we propose that his primary expectation will be that the referral will result in competent treatment and that the specialist has at his disposal, and will employ for the patient's benefit, a professional skill of potential value. At the start of this chapter we pointed out that in the case of psychiatric referrals this professional expectation does not always operate. We suggested that many a psychiatric referral is doomed to failure right at the start because the referring doctor really expects nothing at all or because he expects magical or superhuman results. Both these expectations are a reflection of the referring doctor's inability to see the psychiatrist as a competent peer, and thus with such a doctor there is no way for the psychiatrist to operate in that role. In such situations it is the referring doctor's bias that ensures the psychiatrist's position of alienation; either he sends patients that no one could hope to make better or he sends no patients at all. We like to think that this sort of situation is growing less frequent. As medical schools improve upon the kind of psychiatric exposure that they offer their students, presumably it will lessen the tendency of physicians to view psychiatrists *a priori* as nonpeers and will increase their awareness of the realistic values of psychiatry.

Unfortunately, even where this primary expectation exists, referral relationships all too often go awry. And if there is one single factor that can be fingered for blame, it seems to be the lack of satisfying interprofessional communication, a situation for which the physician tends to see the psychiatrist as totally at fault. To be very specific, we would guess that the biggest complaint by referring doctors is that they do not get what they consider to be adequate written reports from the psychiatrists to whom they refer. They might say that they would even settle for adequate verbal reports but do not seem able to get those either. Having spent several years intimately involved in the psychiatric referral system, we know the frustration experienced by the referring physician over lack of information from the psychiatric consultant. We have seen referring physicians livid with rage at this discourteous oversight on the part of the psychiatrist. There are some valid reasons for the psychiatrist limiting his reports to the referring physician which we shall discuss in detail; however, there is no excuse whatsoever for the psychiatrist failing to acknowledge the referral in writing and perhaps being more explicit by means of a telephone call to the referring physician. After having spent several years training psychiatric residents in a large university outpatient unit where a standing rule directed the residents to write letters to all referring physicians concerning their patients, we are able to state categorically that it is extremely difficult to persuade psychiatric residents to write such letters for the reasons we shall go into later in this chapter. We reiterate, there is no reasonable excuse for the psychiatrist failing to communicate with the referring physician; however, the physician, as we shall attempt to elaborate further, should not expect the same kind of report he receives from his nonpsychiatric consultant.

There is by now a small but very enlightening body of literature discussing the value and meaning of written reports to physicians. The earlier-mentioned study by Bergen at Dartmouth summarizes some of the currently available information on the subject. It may sound naive in the telling of it, but it seems that written reports to one another are a very significant way doctors have of paying their mutual respect to one another. A written report, quite apart from its practical value, carries the unspoken message that the sender sees the receiver as a medical equal, someone with whom it is proper and ethical to discuss patient matters, someone whose professional standing will enable him to understand and use the information being conveyed to him. The very use of technical terms acknowledges a common background and the sharing of medical confidences acknowledges a fraternal relationship.

Lest anyone think we are making much out of nothing, let us share an example having nothing to do with psychiatry at all. The radiation therapy unit at a large university hospital treated for malignancy a patient who, it turned out, had been referred for diagnosis and treatment by a chiropractor. When the patient was ready for discharge, the senior staffman was concerned about the propriety of responding to this nonpeer referral source. He asked the advice of the medical society and received an interesting answer. The society supported his desire to act in the best interests of the patient and of other patients like him and for that reason all agreed that some contact with the chiropractor was desirable. But the society recommended that the contact be via telephone rather than by means of a written letter. Over the phone the radiation therapist could convey the same factual information that would be sent in a letter. But a letter would, they felt, give an extra message that they did not want to send, and that message would be an acknowledgement of a reciprocal professional relationship. Rarely does the symbolic meaning of a referring doctor's written report get spelled out this openly. But we feel that the meaning is operative all the time. And we are proposing that when doctors do not get letters from psychiatrists, they interpret this as a serious breach of medical etiquette and a severe personal put down.

One solution would be for psychiatrists to begin to write the same kind of letter that other doctors write and to supplement them with the same kinds of verbal interchange that other doctors use when talking of patients in whose treatment they share. Unfortunately, this would not be in the best interests of the patients. It is our hope that in sharing with nonpsychiatrists the reasons why psychiatrists communicate with other doctors as they do, their behavior will no longer be seen as obnoxious but rather as part of their fulfillment of the referring physician's basic expectation, namely, that of competent, professional patient care.

A significant part of a psychiatrist's skill is his respect for the patient's communications. Along with this goes a heightened awareness of the impact on the patient of the physician's communications. For example, psychiatrists make hospital rounds very differently from the way that other doctors do. Other doctors talk about their patients right in front of them. Certainly, psychiatrists discuss their patients, but they do not follow the medical tradition of standing at the foot of the bed and talking among themselves as though the patients were not there. A group of psychiatrists would only conduct such a bedside conference if they were including the patient as an actual participant. A prime reason for this is the fact that it is the patient's understanding of himself rather than the psychiatrist's that will be of final therapeutic value. Another equally important reason is that the whole process of psychotherapy is aimed at increasing the patient's sense of personal autonomy; thus he is viewed as an equal, active participant, not as someone to be acted upon by those with greater authority and power than his own.

This philosophy is so basic to most psychiatrists who perform psychotherapy that it inclines them to send very sketchy reports back to referring doctors. They are reluctant to assume the role of talking about their patients, and they would far rather encourage the patients to talk for themselves, to share with the referring doctor whatever they feel they want to share, thus experiencing another area of autonomy in the therapy situation.

Not only is the patient's developing autonomy at stake, so is his need for privacy and dignity. Perhaps no other field of medicine places so high a value on respecting confidentiality. A patient simply needs to know that what he discusses with his therapist will not be disclosed to others unless he, the patient, chooses to do so. It is equally important to be able to assure him that the therapist's assessment of him will not be disclosed without his permission. Perhaps it is here that the competent therapist most blatantly transgresses the classical medical model in relating to a referring doctor. He may demur from using any diagnostic labels and decline to summarize what he sees as "wrong with the patient." Partly this stems from the real inadequacies of our current psychiatric labelling system. Human behavior is so complex and labelling so simplistic that no diagnostic category can completely identify any specific human being. Partly the reluctance to give a diagnosis stems from not wanting to give a sense of permanence to what is hopefully a transient condition or experience and from not wanting to burden someone with a label that may handicap him in the future. For example, the rather benign diagnosis of "anxiety neurosis" really does nothing to increase our understanding of a patient, but it may seriously jeopardize his future insurability.

There is a third factor that helps account for the reticence psychotherapists display when it comes to diagnosing their patients or discussing their psychodynamics. The vocabulary which they use tends to have a different impact on nonpsychiatrists and often sounds far more pathological to them than it does to psychiatrists. For example, a middle aged businessman attains a long hoped for promotion and then begins to experience severe anxiety attacks. He asks his family doctor for the name of a competent psychiatrist and embarks upon a course of psychotherapy. A key issue in his anxiety turns out to be unconscious conflict over homosexual feelings. To psychotherapists who accept the notion that all of us have latent bisexual tendencies, this aspect of the man's conflict presents no particular problem nor does it connote serious pathology. To a general practitioner with a somewhat different orientation, this kind of information might prove very troublesome. And the whole point is that sharing it with the referring doctor would not effectively increase that doctor's understanding of his patient; it would serve no useful purpose at all. Putting such explanations in a written letter would be even worse; such a formulation could only be potentially destructive for the patient.

A second example can demonstrate another situation in which disclosure could be destructive. Once again we shall talk about a patient with anxiety, this time a thirty-year-old housewife whose family doctor refers her because her symptoms have not responded to a brief trial with one of the minor tranquilizers. The doctor receives a brief note from the psychiatrist saying that he and the patient have met and have agreed to begin working together on a twice/week basis. Her husband had been in favor of the evaluation and is now paying for the on-going therapy. He also wants to know what is happening, what is making his wife so anxious and how the therapist is helping and how he, the husband, should behave toward the wife. His concern appears genuine; the family doctor is concerned too. He suggests that the husband contact the psychiatrist whom he may or may not have met as part of the evaluation— Good suggestion, except that a week or so later he calls back to say that he met with the psychiatrist but did not get much satisfaction. The therapist had agreed to see him only after checking with the wife and then only on the condition that the three of them meet together. The husband came away from the encounter with the feeling that he had said quite a bit and that the psychiatrist had said rather little other than that he and the patient were engaged in working together to help her find out who she is and what she wants to be. Now the husband asks the family doctor if he would please call the psychiatrist and see what he can find out; after all the psychiatrist was probably less than totally frank because the patient was sitting right there. As it happens, the immediate cause of the wife's marked anxiety was her recent involvement in an extramarital affair, an experience which produced great guilt but also made her aware of some things that seemed to be lacking in herself and in her marriage. It was not because the patient was sitting there with them that the psychiatrist refrained from relating this to the husband. It was because the question of telling or not telling her husband was one of the issues the patient was in the process of working out in her therapy. Very clearly the decision as well as the disclosure was hers to make, not the therapist's. In the same sense it was not his prerogative to share this information with the family doctor, who really would not be helped by it and whose allegiance was necessarily divided between the spouses as both were his patients.

Because of the three factors we have just been discussing, psychiatrists do not simply struggle with what to tell referring doctors, they have an ever present problem deciding what to put into writing for their own records. Always there is the need to put enough into one's records in order to help one's memory and protect oneself legally and yet there is another need to protect the patient's privacy and dignity should the records ever be ordered into a court of law. The legal concept of privileged communication, which purports to exempt physicians' records from subpoena and thus ensure the patient's privacy, is not operative in all states and even in those states where it is, the exceptions are so numerous as to offer the patient and physician very little protection. As a result it is believed that many psychiatrists keep double records and some try to keep no records at all. We are not here concerning ourselves with the ethics of maintaining confidentiality regarding acts that clearly transgress the law (admitted homocide, for example). We are talking about every day, run-of-the-mill psychiatric observations and formulations that, if read aloud in a court of law, could only be misunderstood and badly distorted.

There are several situations in which the psychiatrist may deal with the referring doctor far more in accordance with the medical model. One is the situation in which a patient requires hospitalization. Here, considerations other than patient privacy will have to take precedence. To begin with, the act of hospitalizing someone indicates that the patient, at least for the present, cannot function autonomously, and that those who are hospitalizing him are assuming some actual responsibility for him. A very essential part of that responsibility is the task of keeping the patient's other caretakers—and this certainly includes the patient's primary physician —informed as to what is going on. This means that following admission, the referring physician ought to get a summarizing letter offering a direct appraisal of the patient's illness and a clear account of what is going to be done as regards a treatment program. Some estimate as to length of hospital stay and expected degree of recovery is also helpful. After the initial report there should be periodic interim reports with the physician receiving advance notice of discharge and a very precise discharge note (citing the patient's maintenance medication, if any, as explicity as it would appear on a prescription pad). From what we have said already about the problems of labelling, it becomes apparent that a real disadvantage to hospitalization is that it will demand that a specific diagnosis be attached to the patient.

A second instance in which the psychiatrist will relate to the referring doctor more nearly like any other physician occurs in the providing of consultation in a general hospital setting. But even here there will be some important distinctions. The psychiatrist will make more of a point of informing the patient as to who he is and why he is there to see the patient. He will make it very clear at the outset that he will be relaying to the referring doctor any material that comes out of the interview, including his own evaluation of the presenting problem and his treatment recommendations. An avowal to the patient that all useful information will be passed on to the requesting doctor is by no means the same as putting it all in the hospital chart where it becomes available to many eyes. Therefore, in order to get full benefit from a hospital consultation, it is often worthwhile to meet per phone or in person with the consultant following the evaluation. It is not that the psychiatrist is too lazy or too uncertain to write it all down; he is exercising professional judgment as to the most constructive mode of communication.

A third situation in which psychiatrists are likely to relate to referring physicians in a manner more nearly like the traditional medical model occurs in those instances in which the psychiatrist tends to employ a preponderance of somatic therapies as opposed to long-term psychotherapy. These practitioners are general psychiatrists who are willing to see very large numbers of patients and are particularly skilled in treating those patients not suited to insight therapy. Their services are, therefore, invaluable to the referring physician and, because of their professional style which more nearly approximates that of the style of nonpsychiatrists, they offer the additional advantage of being far more direct in their responses to those who refer to them.

It has been our aim in this chapter to explain some of the seeming aloofness displayed by those psychiatrists who deal in psychotherapy, and we have focussed on the written report as the paradigm of that seeming aloofness. Before closing we would like to mention several other areas of professional behavior which may well appear to be attempts at isolation, but as with the written report, have good therapeutic reasons behind them.

Psychotherapists are, to begin with, difficult to reach on the telephone. During office hours they usually adhere to uninterruptible schedules. If one wishes to make a referral, he will probably have to put in a call and then wait for a reply. Many therapists, even if they have secretaries, prefer to make their own appointments. Once one has reached the therapist, he may choose not to offer an appointment time at all. Instead, he may ask that the patient contact him directly. When the patient does, the physician may, as already discussed, receive only the briefest letter of acknowledgement. Perhaps the letter may simply state that the patient and therapist have met, that psychotherapy seems suitable, and that it is to begin on a once/week, twice/week (or whatever) schedule. If subsequently the physician visits with the therapist, he may volunteer no progress report at all. Indeed, if the physician asks about the patient, he may offer only the most general statement and refer all other questions back to the patient himself. If the physician tries to share with him information that relatives have passed on to him, the therapist may seem not even to want to hear it.

Therapists cannot respond to phone calls as readily as other physicians because they are providing their patients with a different kind of service. They work with their patients by the hour and not by the symptom or the procedure. Interruptions during the hour would be highly disruptive to the on-going process of therapy. In addition, the mechanics of responding to such calls would be awkward. In other specialties doctors do not seem to hesitate to discuss one patient in the presence of another, and thus, they are comfortable taking calls in their consultation rooms. Psychotherapists, on the other hand, would not want to do this. Therefore, they restrict their telephoning to those few minutes between appointments. Physicians as a group do not like to be kept waiting, and this aspect of a therapist's practice can often be felt as an affront. (Psychiatrists of course, have the same problem in trying to talk with other psychiatrists.)

Often in other practices, a physician will place a referring call for a patient who is still seated in his office and will then get an appointment time for him while he waits. Here again the therapist's reluctance to employ this procedure may seem like a rebuff to the other doctor. It is nothing of the kind. Appointment-making can be an important evaluative tool in psychotherapy, and, thus, the psychiatrist very often prefers talking directly with the patient. Since motivation is one of the very obvious factors to be evaluated, leaving it to the patient to contact the psychiatrist can be a useful procedure.

In summary, we have attempted to delineate some of the expectations which the nonpsychiatric physician has a right to have fulfilled by the psychiatric consultant. We feel it is fair to state that if the referring physician has a comfortable relationship with the consultant prior to the referral, the referral itself and the special communications process involved in the referral will go well. The referring physician should receive appropriate feedback from the consultant, but it is necessary that both consultant and referring physician carefully consider the ground rules concerning the dispersal of this information, so that proper patient care will eventuate.

Chapter VI

SUMMARY

As WE HAVE RELATED in the preceding chapters, the interpersonal relationship between the referring physician and the psychiatric consultant is of extreme importance in caring for one's patients, yet it is one of the most difficult relationships in medicine. It reflects, to a great extent, the professional relationships within medicine on a larger scale. The practice of psychiatry, historically, grew apart from the rest of medicine. Treatment of the mad was often looked upon as a less than worthy endeavor for a physician. Weyer's attack on the institutionalized views of witchcraft made him unpopular with the Church. Dorothea Dix's assault upon the imprisonment and punishment of the mentally ill was resisted by governmental forces. Freud was ostracized from the medical community for his theories of infantile sexuality. Psychiatry, of historical necessity, was forced to withdraw itself from the mainstream of medicine in America. For a long time, it was less than respectable to be interested in mental disorders.

The advent of the somatic therapies heralded a new era in psychiatry and tentative acceptance by medicine in general. Noguchi's isolation of the *Treponema pallidum,* von Jauregg's malarial treatment for general paresis, Sakel's insulin therapy, Cerletti and Bini's discovery of the usefulness of ECT, and, perhaps most importantly, the discovery of the phenothiazines for the psychoses brought psychiatry into closer alignment with other branches of medicine. With the passage of the Community Mental Health Centers Act of

69

1963, the mental health movement became a legitimate and popular area for public support. Yet, the old ambivalence remains. It is "good" to support the ideal of mental health; at the same time, it is "bad" to see a psychiatrist in many areas of this country. One who deals with the unseen psychological forces is often viewed with suspicion and distrust. The fear of the unknown persists.

As psychiatry strives to become more of a scientific discipline acceptable to itself and medicine on the one hand, it cannot sever its relationship to the social sciences and philosophy on the other. One cannot deal with emotional disorders without being sensitive to family disintegration and social situations which produce mental illness. Just as Gorgas and Walter Reed were concerned about the malarial and yellow fever swamps, so are psychiatrists concerned with the breeding sites of social disorder.

The physician may view psychiatry through the distortions of his own intrapsychic conflicts, he may distrust it because of its "liberality" and identification with those involved with social unrest, or he may misconceive it due to faulty training and lack of information. At the same time, psychiatry, which is often overly defensive, may tend to seclude and isolate itself with a false sense of superintellectualization, interest in "humanity," and philosophizing.

Certainly, it behooves the nonpsychiatric physician and the psychiatrist to seek a common ground, if for no other reason than to help their mutual patients. We feel that this common ground can best be achieved in the referral process—by the physicians working together to further the advances of medicine in general.

BIBLIOGRAPHY

1. (The) anatomy of violence. *Roche Medical Image and Commentary, 12*: 22, January, 1970.
2. Bergen, Bernard J.; Weiss, Robert J.; Sanborn, Charlotte J.; and Solow, Charles: Experts and clients: the problem of structural strain in psychiatric consultations. *Diseases of the Nervous System, 31*:396, 1970.
3. Here come the lobotomists again. *Medical World News, 11*:34, January 15, 1971.
4. Hitchcock, E.: Psychosurgery today. *Annals of Clinical Research, 3*:187, 1971.
5. Kalinowsky, Lothar: The convulsive therapies. *Comprehensive Textbook of Psychiatry*, Alfred Freeman and Harold Kaplan, ED., Baltimore, Williams and Wilkins Company, 1970, pp. 1279-1285.
6. Kimsey, Larry R.: Mental health commitment in Dallas County. *Dallas Medical Journal, 54*:381, 1968.
7. Kimsey, Larry R. and Titone, Anita M.: Use of mental health volunteers. *Dallas Medical Journal, 55*:543, 1969.
8. Kimsey, Larry R. and Frost, Mary: Long term camping for emotionally disturbed boys. *Diseases of the Nervous System, 32*:35, January, 1971.
9. Koegler, Ronald R.; Hicks, Shelby M.; and Barger, James H.: Medical and psychiatric use of electrosleep. *Diseases of the Nervous System, 32*:100, 1971.
10. Liddon, Sim C.: The referring physician and the psychiatric consultant. *Postgraduate Medicine, 51*:179, 1972.
11. Mariner, Allen S.: Psychotherapists' communications with patients' relatives and referring professionals. *American Journal of Psychotherapy, 25*:517, October, 1971.
12. Piedmont, Eugene B.: Referrals and reciprocity: psychiatrists, general practitioners, and clergymen. *Journal of Health and Social Behavior, 9*:29, March, 1968.
13. Scanlan, John M.: Physician to student: the crisis of psychiatric residency training. *The American Journal of Psychiatry, 128*:1107, 1972.
14. Study disputes charges of over-prescribing by physicians. *Psychiatric News, 7*:13, May 3, 1972.
15. Tischler, Gary L.: The transition into residency. *The American Journal of Psychiatry, 128*:1103, 1972.
16. Weiner, Myron F.: Asking the psychiatrist for help . . . helpful hints to the referring physician. *Texas State Journal of Medicine, 61*:488, 1965.

CONTENTS

73